BECOMING
BOSTON
STRONG

BECOMING BOSTON STRONG

One Woman's Race to Run and Conquer the World's Greatest Marathon

Amy Noelle Roe

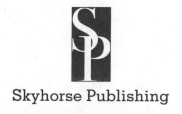

Skyhorse Publishing

Skyhorse Publishing books may be purchased in bulk at special discounts for sales promotion, corporate gifts, fund-raising, or educational purposes. Special editions can also be created to specifications. For details, contact the Special Sales Department, Skyhorse Publishing, 307 West 36th Street, 11th Floor, New York, NY 10018 or info@skyhorsepublishing.com.

Skyhorse® and Skyhorse Publishing® are registered trademarks of Skyhorse Publishing, Inc.®, a Delaware corporation.

Visit our website at www.skyhorsepublishing.com.

10 9 8 7 6 5 4 3 2

Library of Congress Cataloging-in-Publication Data is available on file.

Cover design by Paul Qualcom
Cover photo credit: iStockphoto

Print ISBN: 978-1-5107-4205-5
Ebook ISBN: 978-1-5107-4170-6

Printed in the United States of America.

CONTENTS

· · · · · · · · · ·

"Running, one might say, is basically an absurd pastime upon which to be exhausting ourselves. But if you can find meaning in the type of running you need to do . . . chances are you'll be able to find meaning in that other absurd pastime—life."

—Bill Bowerman

PROLOGUE: APRIL 17, 2013

A BOOM ECHOES throughout downtown. Another one follows. Looking west down Boylston Street, I see a plume of smoke rising between the buildings.

At mile 21 of the Boston Marathon, at the crest of the infamous Heartbreak Hill, Boston College students had erected a giant inflatable arch that triumphantly declared, "The heartbreak is over."

Now, blocks from the finish line of the 117th Boston Marathon, I sense the heartbreak is only beginning.

My hands are cold; my stomach is in knots. A shiver of fear runs through my body. Moments ago, I was relieved to be handed my gear-check bag, which had been misplaced. When it finally turned up, I swaddled myself in warm, dry clothes, comforted by the fact that finally I'd done what I set out to do, and in the way that I'd wanted to do it.

I'm not a talented athlete. This is not false modesty; it's a cold, hard fact. I didn't take up running until I was thirty-one, and at first, I was so self-conscious that I would only jog at night, hoping that no one I knew would see me. Running was hard enough; I didn't need the added pressure of an audience. Whenever I tried to run I was so uncomfortable that I imagined one would need a will of iron to force themselves to do it for long.

Still, to move through space with no help from anyone or anything seemed to me like the ultimate in independence and self-determination. And, outdoors, in the fresh air, was where I'd always felt most at peace.

So, while the activity of running didn't feel natural, it became for me increasingly aspirational, a way to bridge the gaping chasm between who I felt I was and who I hoped to be. I thought of runners as indomitable people, way out of my league. But I figured if I completed a marathon maybe I could call myself a runner, too.

Over the course of a few months I worked up the courage to run in the full light of day, but it took ten marathons over the next five years before I covered 26.2 miles fast enough to qualify for the Boston Marathon. And then it seemed that I was cursed; three weeks before my non-refundable flight to Boston, an injury threatened to dash my dream of even starting the race.

My foot in a walking cast with the 2011 Boston Marathon three weeks away—this felt like hell to me, or at least a kind of purgatory. It was like I was the ill-fated heroine in some black comedy. But to see myself as the protagonist in a story gave me some much-needed perspective so in my head I began to write that story, not knowing how it would end.

Stories had always come easy to me. I'd spent more than a decade as a newspaper reporter and editor. Stories were how I paid the bills, but journalists are expected to be objective, to put a professional distance between themselves and the subject. In the newsrooms where I cut my reporter teeth, writing in the first person was strongly discouraged.

"You," an editor once told me pointedly, "are not the story."

After crossing the finish line of the 2013 Boston Marathon, I leaned against a yellow school bus, exhausted but elated, and pulled track pants over my shivering body. I had spent years working towards earning a spot at Boston. Yet I was totally unprepared for what happened next, for the way that, in a matter of minutes, history seemed to be rising up all around me.

After the bombs exploded, I found myself in a breaking news event—one that I was experiencing, rather than covering. I was not the story, far from it. But as I told reporters what I'd seen and heard, I sensed a larger narrative unfolding, one that began years earlier and would carry on long beyond the tragedy on Boylston Street.

CHAPTER ONE

Heartbreak

I AM CAUGHT in a crowd of runners shuffling feebly through the streets when my cell phone rings. My dad's raspy voice is on the other end: "Amy?"

He has no idea what had just happened. He can't know. No one, save for those of us who have just seen and heard the explosions, knows about this yet.

"Yes, Dad. It's Amy. I'm okay, Dad. I'm here in Boston. There's been an accident, but I'm okay."

A white lie. One look at the smoke that swirls up the side of the buildings and I know this is no accident and that deep down, I am far from okay.

"When are you coming?" Dad asks. This is the first thing he says when he calls me, which is on average five or six times a day—sometimes more if I don't pick up. We always have the same short conversation, as if following a script. Dad either doesn't remember where I am and what I am doing, or he simply hasn't given it a thought.

"I'm coming on Wednesday," I say. "I'll see you Wednesday, okay?"

"Okay," he mumbles and hangs up.

I snap my phone shut and keep on shuffling. This conversation comes as no surprise. Back in Seattle, my dad is recovering from a series of small strokes he suffered two weeks earlier. He lives alone, and a neighbor found him in his house and called 911. For once, Dad had been unable to refuse an ambulance. He was treated in the hospital's stroke

1

unit and transferred to another facility for rehab a couple of days before I left for Boston.

My running coach, in his emailed instructions, said in the week leading up to the race I should avoid stress and focus on "peaking." But I am the only person responsible for my Dad; my siblings both live far away. The week has been a flurry of phone calls to doctors, social workers, and family members to arrange for my dad's care. All the while, I'd felt guilty for fearing his latest crisis might keep me from getting to Boston and for wanting to come here and run instead of staying with him.

At the moment, part of me feels I should say something to both my dad and the stream of strangers coming toward me, to warn them about what I have just seen, but what would I say? *Don't freak out, but I think there was just a bombing?*

It is pointless to try to explain. The Red Sox fans milling about after today's game are sure to encounter pandemonium if they keep walking downtown. And my dad will eventually turn on CNN.

Marathon volunteers clad in bright yellow jackets urge me and my fellow runners to walk away from the direction of the smoke, which is now billowing into the sky. As I follow their instructions, it occurs to me that the people streaming toward me are as oblivious as my seventy-eight-year-old father in a nursing home on the other side of the country. At this point, only a small number people—just those of us in the immediate vicinity of the explosions—have any inkling of what is happening. Realizing I am among them fills me with dread. This is one exclusive club I don't want to be in.

People clad in red and blue are coming toward me, which confirms I'm heading toward Fenway Park, and the Howard Johnson Fenway Inn, where my husband, Daniel, and I are staying. I realize I need to find a way over the Mass Pike, the freeway that cuts through the city, in order to get there, but I don't know where to cross it.

A crowd gathers outside a dry cleaner, watching a television through the window. I start to shuffle across the street toward them, but something makes me stop. I know from covering news events as a reporter that details of the explosions will be slow in coming, but in the meantime, there'll be an abundance of fear and speculation, two things of no use to me. Stopping to watch would be unhelpful.

What I need is to see Daniel again.

I had my phone in my hand, about to call him, when I hear the second explosion.

"Just get out of there," I said as soon as he answered, referring to a corner outside the Hynes Convention Center, near the finish line, where we'd planned to meet. We agreed to meet back at the hotel instead. To do that, I can't just stand here and watch TV. Pulling my foil post-race blanket around me against the breeze, I continue shuffling in the direction of the HoJo.

My legs are stiff. So many people are coming toward me and no one yields, so I expend energy that I really don't have weaving around them, like a fish desperately attempting to swim upstream. The fact that I have just finished the marathon apparently means nothing; they have places to go.

But one man stops and looks me square in the face. He says something to me, but it's as if someone has turned the volume way down. My world is on mute.

"Excuse me?" I say.

"ARE . . . YOU . . . OKAY?" he repeats, practically shouting now.

I am not sure how to answer. I am alone on the streets of Boston, exhausted, confused, bereft. Some bombs have gone off—of that I am certain—and I have no idea what might happen next. Okay is hardly how I would describe myself right now.

But I can barely register my emotions, let alone explain them to a stranger. "Yes," I say, finally. "Thank you."

I walk a couple more blocks before I realize my answer is a massive overstatement, if not a flat-out lie. In fact, I am trembling, dangerously low on the adrenaline that has gotten me this far, and yet so oblivious to my condition that I did not even recognize the man's question for what it is: an offer of help.

Help, I realize, is exactly what I need, so I begin to look around for anyone who can provide it.

As I make my way past a motel parking lot, I hear some young women yelling to each other from a distance. Someone says something about Kenmore Square. I turn and look at them. "Are you going to Kenmore Square?" I ask, desperation creeping into my voice. They must also see the urgency on my face, drained of its color.

"Do you need a ride?" the nearer of the two replies. They are dressed in a preppy, East Coast-style that reminds me of girls I knew in college, from the women's colleges of Smith and Mount Holyoke. This shred of familiarity is oddly comforting to me.

I reply that if they are going that way, I would appreciate a ride. I can feel myself choking up as I speak; I am beyond grateful.

Don't cry, I tell myself. *You'll scare away the preppies.*

A few moments later I am in a burgundy SUV with a man I've never met behind the wheel. I have never been so relieved to get inside a car with strangers; I nearly kneel and kiss the upholstery. We introduce ourselves quickly, but their names evaporate almost immediately from my fatigued mind. The girls are all on their smartphones, trying to connect with a friend who had been running the race when it was called off. Volunteers diverted her to side streets near Kenmore Square, and they're not sure where she is right now. I explain that I finished the marathon but got separated from my husband, who returned to our hotel to wait for me. No one asks any more questions after that, and I'm glad.

Taking out my flip phone, I first text Dan: "Some nice girls are giving me a ride," and then I start to look at my other messages.

One of the text messages I receive is from a friend who works at an NPR affiliate in Seattle. She wants me to do an interview with a reporter who is covering the aftermath of the bombings in real time. I text back my agreement, and minutes later, my phone is ringing. When I answer the call, the reporter puts me on the air live and asks me what I've seen.

"I heard a big boom coming from that direction. We all turned and looked, then we heard another boom, and there was a huge cloud of smoke," I recall. "At that point, you know, no one knew what was going on, but race volunteers started telling us to disperse and get away down the other side of the street. So that's what I did."

The reporter asks me how I'd characterize the explosions.

"It looked like something nefarious; it didn't look like something that was accidental," I say.

Daniel and I often jokingly refer to "nefarious activity" to describe shady goings-on in our neighborhood, but this is the first time I've ever used the word with someone else, in serious conversation. The reporter, unfazed by my word choice, asks me how others reacted.

"We had just run a marathon, so we were just . . . I don't think people, immediately, were panicking. But they were definitely shocked," I say. "There was a little bit of a pause, and then you started to hear all the sirens. And we were just very worried, and . . . it got kind of chaotic."

When the reporter asks me how I am feeling, I nearly break down.

"I was planning to meet my husband near the finish line, and fortunately, he was not in the area. But there was a moment when I thought, you know . . ." My voice starts cracking.

I regain a bit of composure. "I looked down the street and looked at where we were supposed to meet, and until I heard his voice, I was just terrified."

The reporter thanks me for my time, and after I get off the phone, I feel shaken up all over again. I have with me the small bag of food they give you after you cross the finish line, so I rummage through it, ready to eat my feelings. None of the food appeals to me (*Why isn't there chocolate?*), but I know I should consume some calories. It might make me feel better. I tear off some pieces of a King's Hawaiian sweet roll and chew mechanically, washing down the dry bread with swigs of bottled water.

My phone rings again. This time the voice is familiar. On the line is Brian Calvert, a radio journalist at a media company where I used to work. With him on the other line was Daniel; it's the first I've spoken to him since our brief conversation seconds after the bombs exploded. It is good to hear Brian's kind, calm baritone, and even better when I get to hear my husband again.

Dan tells Brian he was about a block away from the explosions. When asked to describe them, Dan is uncharacteristically blunt: "It was a big fireball," he says. Brian notes that authorities are careful not to call it a bomb.

"What I know of a bomb," Dan says, "it looked like a bomb to me."

Brian asks me how I'm doing. I'm still reeling from the news that my husband had been in the vicinity of a "big fireball," but I try to sound composed.

"Oh, I'm fine. I'm obviously a bit shaken up, but I'm fine. I was on Boylston Street, but several blocks down. I heard a loud explosion, an incredibly loud boom, then I saw this long cloud of smoke. I just saw a huge amount of smoke. It looked like some kind of bomb or something, it was huge."

"Did any of you get a number of . . ." Brian says, trailing off. But I know what he means.

"I haven't heard any reports of any fatalities at this point," I say.

Moments later, my phone drops the call. I can hear the dial tone over the air. I snap it shut.

Now I realize my heart is pounding. I sit back in the car and try to relax. I don't mind that the interview has ended, except that it has also severed my connection to Dan.

I keep texting Dan updates, informing him when we stop for gas. Mostly, I just want to keep our line of communication open and to have the reassurance he is okay. Finally, after about half an hour of driving, we are in an area I recognize, and I ask to be let out of the vehicle to walk. Thanking everyone in the car, I hobble onto the street, gimpy after sitting down for so long. Other runners who had not finished the race when it was called off are making their way along the streets. I find myself ambling stiff-legged alongside a silver-haired man who says he had been stopped while on the course, and from his grave expression I get the distinct impression he knows exactly why.

We make eye contact and shake our heads in mutual disbelief. "The Boston Marathon?" I say, incredulous.

"Is nothing sacred?" he replies, equally stunned.

I continue walking, and at long last I reach the Howard Johnson motel. From the pocket of my shorts I take out the motel room key card that I have carried more than twenty-seven miles. I fumble with it for only a moment before Dan flings open the door. I'll never forget the intense look on his face before he hugs me tightly to him. We just stand there in silence. I close my eyes and breathe in the smell of him, grateful we are both alive and, at last, together.

In the bathroom, I strip off my clothes. Reflected in the shabby mirror, my face looks haggard and pale. How I have aged since the morning! My back stings; It's pink where I missed applying sunscreen. There is a red slash across my torso, where my sports bra has rubbed my skin raw. My feet are swollen, my toes tender. I can tell that under the dark metallic nail polish I painted on them, a couple of toenails are bruised black, goners for sure.

After most marathons, I take an ice bath, but it is several hours too late to be optimizing my recovery. I stand under the shower, warm water stinging me as it washes the salt from my skin. Blood from my chafed skin swirls down the drain. Blood, sweat, and tears, I think to myself. I just haven't gotten to the last part, yet.

Drying off, my skin feels hypersensitive, as if all my nerve endings are firing at once. The cheap hotel towel might as well be sandpaper. I put on the softest clothes I have with me and microwave the white box that contains leftovers of my pre-race pasta dinner. News coverage on TV makes it clear the explosions have now officially been classified as bombings.

I struggle to eat the rest of my pasta. It had been delicious just hours ago. Now I barely taste the forkfuls I shovel into my mouth. I can tell I am dehydrated, so I drink Gatorade and water, all the while keeping my eyes glued to the television.

"Here's how you know some crazy shit has just gone down," I say to Dan as I flip through the seemingly infinite cable channels. Every one of them shows the exact same image: a somber President Obama making a statement. For perhaps the first time in my life, I feel a deep personal interest in what the president is saying. I hang on every word. At long last we have something to talk about, but the conversation only goes in one direction.

"We still do not know who did this or why, and people shouldn't jump to conclusions before we have all the facts," Obama tells reporters. "But make no mistake, we will get to the bottom of this. We will find out who did this, we will find out why they did this. Any responsible individuals, any responsible groups, will feel the full weight of justice."

The full weight of justice. It is as if President Obama is speaking to me directly through the hotel's ancient tube television, informing me in his calm, measured way that the government will do its job and that my job is to be patient.

The sounds fair, but fair isn't what I want to hear right now. Nothing else about today has been fair. Instead, I want the president to sound angry, to be as outraged as me, to seem a little more on "our" side. But whose "side" is that? We have no idea who is responsible.

Now it hits me: Not even the Leader of the Free World can fix this. It's a chilling thing to comprehend.

For the next couple hours, Dan and I continue emailing and texting and watching news reports, manically shifting attention between big and small screens. We learn that two people are confirmed dead. I fear the death toll will only grow. Dan works for a Seattle television news station, so he called into the newsroom as soon as he'd reached me on the phone earlier; he's spoken to a few outlets thus far. I hear him do a couple more interviews on the phone as I speak to some friends and family members. I down a can of Coke from the machine; the caffeine seems to loosen my headache's vise grip.

Our small hotel room is in disarray. Clothes, towels, and cell phone chargers are strewn about pell-mell. We have to get out of here.

For one thing, we both need more to eat. We need to leave our room to find food, but with the perpetrators still at large, what place is safe?

Leaving also means I need to get dressed. And that raises another heavy question: What to wear?

On a typical race day, the answer is easy. For many, if not most marathoners, it is a tradition to change into a race shirt and/or finisher's medal after cleaning up from the race. At Boston, the Boston Marathon jacket is de rigueur post-race. Adidas has made a Boston Marathon jacket, in a different color scheme each year, for twenty-seven years now. The $110 garment is sold at the pre-race expo and online months prior to the race, and purchasing it is a ritual for race participants. Adidas calls it the Celebration Jacket.

But there will be no celebrating today. The jacket, the medal; now I'm not sure what—if anything—these mementoes mean. Still, I remember the response after 9/11, when many people spoke of the importance of "not being cowed" by violence. At the time, it didn't occur to me to question that, but now I'm not sure why it is so terrible to be cowed by violence. Isn't that a normal human survival instinct?

Since I traveled to Boston with only a carry-on backpack, I don't have a lot of options. In fact, as a returning Boston Marathoner, much of the clothing I brought has the Boston Marathon logo on it. Finally, I find myself looping the finisher's medal around my neck and slipping the jacket on over it, just as I did after finishing the 2011 Marathon. It isn't defiance, only protocol. With a rueful smile, I remember the old runners' rule: "Nothing new on race day."

News reports inform us that downtown Boston is on "lockdown," so those staying in the area can't even leave their hotels. Those of us at the Howard Johnson are far enough from the finish line that we are outside of this zone. Across the street from our hotel, a crowd of people spills out of a bar called Sweet Caroline's, named for the Neil Diamond song that's a staple at Red Sox games. It is hard to tell whether the bar patrons are celebrating the Red Sox win or if they have banded together in the wake of tragedy. Either way, I am awed at their camaraderie.

"Damn, Boston," I say to Daniel, in reverent disbelief of what I am seeing. We agree that in a similar scenario in Seattle, the streets would probably be empty, but in this town, people apparently haven't gotten the memo that they are supposed to be cowering in their homes.

The restaurant we had planned to go was closed, so we go to a nearby Chipotle and have tacos. In some places Chipotle serves margaritas, but to my disappointment, this isn't one of them.

A couple of people, seeing my jacket, congratulate me, but unlike when I ran Boston in 2011, there is something awkward and unspoken in their smiles, and in mine in return. My Marathon jacket and their acknowledgement of it—it's like we're only going through the motions now, carrying on amid tragedy and uncertainty because what else can we do?

After we finish eating, I am still craving a salty margarita and after walking for a bit, Daniel and I happen on a Mexican restaurant that is, incongruously, playing 1980s pop music. The televisions are on and showing news footage, while songs from *The Breakfast Club* soundtrack fill the air. I get my margarita, salt encrusted around the rim. Dan has a beer. A nearby table is full of friends stranded in the city. The trains aren't running, so they can't get home. Instead, they seem to be killing time, hanging out drinking. We get to talking. One guy tells me cab drivers are price-gouging. It reminds me of hurricanes and other natural disasters when stores jack up the prices of bottled water.

One of the people at the table is a young woman who was half a mile from the finish line when she was forced to stop running. Police and volunteers halted the race by forming a human chain across the street. It is her first Boston Marathon. She can't stop crying. Concerned, I ask one of her friends how I can help.

"Do you have an extra finisher's medal?" he says.

I doubt she wants a finisher's medal from a race she hasn't finished, especially Boston. The medal's only value is the accomplishment it symbolizes. That is something no one can give her now, and something that can never be taken from me. The woman's friend probably isn't a runner, or he would've realized this.

Still, I don't need my medal. It is just a thing. I exchange glances with Daniel, walk over to the table and kneel beside the young woman, whose pale skin is red from the sun.

The medal now feels heavy in my hand as I offer it to her. A tear streams down her pretty face as she shakes her head no. She says she appreciates it, but she can't take it.

I don't blame her. I would decline the offer, too, were I in her running shoes.

Walking back to our table, I think of something else to console her: "The BAA (Boston Athletic Association, which puts on the race) will invite all of those who didn't finish back to do the race again," I say.

Of this I'm so certain that my voice cracks with emotion. It's the right thing to do, and I am confident race organizers will do it.

I tell her: "You'll be back."

CHAPTER TWO

Soft Targets

APRIL 18, 2013, the day after, dawns with unseemly spring magnificence. Pink blossoms gild the trees that line Beacon Hill's narrow streets, and swans glide in the pond at the Public Garden, same as they have every day following the last 117 Marathon Mondays.

This is what the experts call cognitive dissonance. It's also déjà vu. One morning more than a decade ago on the Gulf Coast of Florida, I awoke to the same uncanny feeling. We were in the middle of a relentless, deadly storm season. I had spent the night alone in my dark, concrete-block apartment; the wind had knocked out the power. Outside, Hurricane Georges raged, ripping off roofs and uprooting trees. I was talking with my sister, Melissa, when my phone, a landline, went dead. Somehow, hunkered down with a bottle of gin, I finally fell asleep. The next morning, I woke up with a splitting headache. The gin had done its job, but sloppily. Daybreak was dissonant. Birds chirped, and the air breathed the scent of magnolias, as if the previous evening had only been a bad dream. When a co-worker from the newspaper where I worked at the time picked me up in his old Jeep, we toured the twisted metal and brutalized buildings on the way to work.

Now, emerging from the Fenway HoJo, approaching the aftermath of what is officially a bombing, I have the same surreal feeling. As we walk down Boylston toward the city center, nearly every business we see is closed, some with hand-written signs on their doors. The streets are cordoned off even blocks away, so we turn around and walk back toward Kenmore Square, towards a bagel shop we passed earlier.

It's open.

As we enter, I do a double take at a National Guardsman walking by. He looks like he's dressed for a war zone in camouflage fatigues, a tan helmet, and an enormous rifle slung over one shoulder. It's as if we are in some post-apocalyptic movie, set in a city under martial law.

Is the world now out of control? Do we need to be wearing Kevlar vests just to secure an everything bagel?

If it looks bad outside the bagel shop, Boston may appear even worse on national news. If our family and friends are seeing National Guardsmen with automatic weapons walking the streets, they're probably freaking out.

But should they be worried? More to the point, should we?

Getting back, the lobby of the Howard Johnson Fenway Inn is bustling, with people desperately trying to get out. We move into the mob.

As we near the front of the check-out line, two men enter the lobby, an older man with what looks to be his younger partner. The older man ignores the long line and goes up to the front desk: "FBI." He startles the clerk by telling him he needs to look at some rooms.

Flustered, the young employee can barely find the words to reply, but FBI guy doesn't give him much time. As if to pre-empt any possible objection, he takes out a badge and holds it up next to his face.

"Keys to the city, right here," he declares.

This is straight out of a movie, maybe a buddy action flick, what with the young buck/veteran agent partnership and badge-flashing bravado.

Now, when we had first arrived, the clerk had remarked that a scene from a movie called *The Town* was filmed in the hotel, in a room not far from the one in which we were staying. I hadn't seen the movie, but I'd heard of it—a Ben Affleck cop drama with Blake Lively as the requisite love interest. From the ads I recalled the *Gossip Girl* star had ditched her Park Avenue style for blue eyeliner and big, gold-hoop earrings; Hollywood code for trashy.

With the appearance of the FBI men, I have to wonder, *Is this a case of life imitating art?*

I smirk to myself at the coincidence. Daniel and I share a look. Neither of us has any interest in staying to see how this movie ends. We hurry through check-out, pocket the claims check for our bags, and step outside.

There are hours before we need to go to the airport. What now? The day after Marathon Monday is usually a joyous occasion. When I'd booked the flight, I'd built in the time because I figured we'd be reluctant to leave and would want to savor the last hours of our Boston Marathon experience. Now I can't wait to go home.

We decide that the best way to waste time is to keep moving. We walk over to a bike-sharing station, swipe a credit card, and set out on heavy city bikes. Following a marked bike route, we pedal east down Commonwealth Avenue, toward the public garden. It feels odd riding a bike without a helmet, but it is also liberating. Normally I'm so safety minded. After everything that has happened over the last thirty-six hours, I've got nothing to lose.

As we approach, we see that a row of white television trucks lines the boulevard. People are wearing Boston Marathon jackets in various colors, each hue signifying a different year. Are they doing this in solidarity? A few carry yellow gear-check bags, probably coming back from a gear-check set up because it was disrupted yesterday.

At the public garden, some runners are passing by. At the sight of my 2013 Boston Marathon jacket, they cheer in unison. I notice many others wearing their Marathon gear, too. The mood seems lighter than last night.

But everywhere are reminders. At the statehouse, a reporter for a Japanese television station stands beneath the golden dome, gazing intently into a camera. Maybe he is reporting live; the world is watching Boston now.

As we arrive in the North End, Daniel powers up the hill on the heavy bike. I keep downshifting, but the bike has few gears. My legs can barely move the pedals. What was supposed to be an easy spin is turning out to be more than I'd bargained for.

"I'm turning around," I yell to him.

My legs ache, they aren't working properly, and I'm angry. Angry at my legs. Angry at this awkward, heavy bike-share bike and at Daniel for making me ride it.

How dare the sky shine so blue and beautiful now? I'm outraged that the trees, with their frilly pink blossoms, rudely refuse to acknowledge that today is any different than yesterday.

Yesterday, did I dream it? I'm a worst-case scenario thinker but the day's events are beyond even my morbid imagination.

No, we have very few facts, including who orchestrated this event and why they did it. Competent, disciplined individuals, the best and the brightest among our nation's civilian and military agencies, are hurriedly pursuing the answers so that no one else gets hurt. In the meantime, all Dan and I can do is turn the pedals on our stupid bikes. It's beyond words how frustrating it is.

Something else is angering me, something I dare not put into words, even to Daniel. That violence interrupted the Boston Marathon—of all major events—which deeply offends me. The Boston Marathon is an event entirely innocent of politics. Until now, only positive words have been associated with it. It is uncontroversial, peaceful, secular, nonpartisan, full of unity and goodwill. The weekend surrounding the Boston Marathon is the distance running equivalent of high holy days. Runners work and prepare, sometimes for years, to bring them about. Our friends and family support us in our efforts, learn about it, hear about it, and ask about it. And because by qualifying one earns the right to participate, being able to compete in it is a rite of passage.

But now violence has marred all of it. And yet, because this harm is nothing compared to the tragic loss others are experiencing, I feel that I don't have the right to speak about this aloud. To do so would be selfish and offensive.

I'm sure I'm not the only one who feels this way, though. No one, I notice, utters the names Lelisa Desisa and Rita Jeptoo, who only yesterday crossed the finish line as champions. Perpetrators of violence blotted out history. Now that it is the site of terror, will the Boston Marathon ever be just a marathon again?

A line from a poem read at my college graduation pops into my mind: "Vietnam is not a war."

It's been years since I heard these words. I get a chill as I recite to myself what little I remember. The poem is about refusing to allow one's identity to be defined by violence. The voice in which it is written is powerful, defiant. But it is not my voice, not even close.

I am in Massachusetts, one of America's original colonies, and what comes to mind is a poem about the legacy of an American war on a peoples' identity. To connect the two: Is it shameful? Am I delusional?

A poem contains no facts, only feelings. This one was written by Lê Thị Diễm Thúy, a student whose family came to the States from Vietnam. She read it at my graduation at Hampshire College. When I heard her words, they were a revelation and a reproach. To my callow American mind, the word war had always followed Vietnam; the two were inextricably linked. The poem forced me to consider the shadow that history casts over the lives of innocent individuals.

My graduation was a nontraditional ceremony; no caps or gowns. Borrowing a tradition from nearby women's colleges, I wore all white, like a suffragette. I listened to the poem, was moved by it, and then happily traipsed in strappy sandals across the grass and into the privileges of adulthood.

To feel safe, to do what I want, to run fearlessly alone or among thousands is not a hobby. It's a right to which all of us are born, simply because we are human.

The emotion this poem evokes for me, then as now, is no less real for my distance from its meaning. Vietnam is not a war. The Boston Marathon is not a bombing. And grief and anger aren't facts, they are feelings.

Maybe, the world over, they feel the same to everybody.

CHAPTER THREE

The Start Line

My marathon story begins ten years earlier and 2,000 miles away. It starts in the city of Portland, Oregon, with me just trying to put one foot in front of the other.

I am not an Oregon native—I'm originally from Seattle, just up Interstate 5, but a job as a staff writer for an alternative weekly has brought me to this West Coast hipster mecca. Once I signed a check at a downtown store, and the clerk glanced at my signature and said, "Amy Roe . . . the writer?"

I am surprised by this recognition and not naïve enough to let it go to my head. If, at thirty years old, I'm mistaken for a big fish, it's only because Portland is a little pond. Lots of people read the paper I write for, and since the staff is small, my name is on the cover approximately every third week.

A few of my pieces get people talking, and it seems I'm in on the rise, "one to watch," as one of those cheesy city magazines say. But staff writers are only as good as our last cover stories. My misses eventually outnumber my hits. My average goes down, and before long, I am out, in a manner so smooth and yet so abrupt that I'm not quite sure what is happening.

They like me. They think I am smart. And I yet I won't be coming back to work on Monday.

This is, of course, not at all how I'd envisioned things when I'd packed up my Jetta a little over a year ago. Portland was supposed to be a stepping stone. But I haven't just slipped on my stepping stone, I've wiped out on it, in front of an entire city. *Now what am I supposed to do?*

For starters, I try: nothing. I make no plans to move from Portland. For the first time in years, I make no plans whatsoever. I am demoralized, and I just want to disappear, and Lloyd Center, the local mall, is the perfect place to do this. It is only a couple miles from my dirt-cheap studio apartment, but it might as well be another world.

My neighborhood is the sort of anti-capitalist hipster enclave satirized by the comedy *Portlandia*. People walk down the street in fuzzy slippers, if they wear shoes at all, carrying their own, hand-thrown ceramic coffee mug into Stumptown Coffee for a refill of drip. Street kids sit on the sidewalk, spanging (spare-changing) and rolling their own cigarettes. Nobody seems in a hurry, maybe because everybody seems a bit stoned.

Lloyd Center is an entirely different scene, or rather, an anti-scene. There isn't a hipster in sight, just a few mall-walking seniors and the requisite scowling teens. Bright, generic, anonymous, it is Anywhere, USA, which is all I require—Anywhere (But Here).

In my junk mail a few days prior, I got a coupon for Jamba Juice, which just happens to have a Lloyd Center location. While waiting for my raspberry-strawberry smoothie with a complimentary power C shot, I notice a flyer about a local marathon training group. Like Jamba Juice, such a pursuit feels very antithetical to my Northeast Portland neighborhood, its inherent optimism serves as a balm to my dark mood.

People have been telling me things will start cooking if only I stop standing over the proverbial pot, willing it to boil. I realize they might be right, but it isn't so easy to shut off my mind. I need something to distract me: Something cheap, but not worthless, to fill my time. If life is what happens to you while you're making other plans, I need some sort of plan, in order to get a life.

So I take a flyer.

Upon further consideration, running a marathon doesn't sound all that fun, actually, and my life is un-fun enough already. Plus, I'm hesitant to take up something new in Portland when I'm not sure how long I'll be around. But I keep picking up the flyer, staring at it, then setting it facedown again on my kitchen table. I can't deny my curiosity. Going that far, all by oneself, must be a powerful feeling. And wouldn't it be nice to feel powerful right now?

A week after that fateful day at Jamba Juice, I show up to run two miles on a bike path along the Willamette River. The marathon-training group is open to anyone, and the two-mile trial run is just to get a sense of which group you should run in. Still, to me, it feels serious, like an audition or a job interview.

Organizers tell us to run "comfortably hard." Instead, I run all-out, passing as many people as I can on the out-and-back route, drawing deep, jagged breaths that probably startle those around me, who do not appear to be taking it nearly as seriously. Maybe I throw an elbow or two. All the while, I try to pretend I am taking it easy, going so casual, dude.

My appearance gives lie to this. When I finish, flushed and gasping, my cotton t-shirt is damp with sweat. The two-mile run takes me sixteen minutes. The number is significant. It means I am assigned to the green group.

We weren't informed beforehand about the eventual sorting into the color-coded groups, so for those running around me, green has no meaning. For whatever reason (curiosity, pride, and fear are likely candidates) I bother to suss out a hierarchy before I even set off on the run. I discern that the green group is not the fastest group, but it is not the slowest, either. In the middle works for me.

The slowest group is the red group; red like a stop sign. Red like emergency—the emergency being that you are in danger of being mistaken for a walker.

I don't want to be in the red group. Better dead than red. When someone hands me a green reflective tag to attach to my shoe, I fasten it to my laces immediately. Green is good. Green means go.

The green tag will stay there for the life of my shoes. I plan to transfer the tag to my new pair if these wear out. Green is my guarantee I won't be in the caboose group. I realize right away that I am not going to win any races, but I sure don't want to come in last.

Satisfied with my penultimate group status, I write a check and join the marathon training program, Portland Fit. The name has a nice ring to it, like getting in shape isn't just good for one's self, that it is also a civic duty. As citizen-runners, we are pounding the pavement in the name of our Rose City.

The membership fee includes a training schedule that runs all the way to race day. Portland Fit is the one place where someone, mercifully, is telling me exactly what to do and when to do it. With no job, set schedule, or sense of what the future holds, my life is utterly lacking in clear instructions or directions, so this feels like a blessing. And the outcome of my effort, though not guaranteed, is strongly implied. If I follow instructions, I will be able to run the Portland Marathon in October 2004. All this for $125? Sounds like a bargain.

Portland Fit doesn't cost much, but it requires a different kind of investment: sweat equity. On Saturday mornings, our group assembles to listen to coaches give tips on items like stretching and nutrition. Then we gather in our color-coded groups and set off along the Willamette River Trail, heading in different directions depending on the length of our assigned runs.

One day I find myself jogging alongside a barrel-chested man with calves like tree trunks. When he learns I'm new to Portland Fit and to running in general, he welcomes me heartily, chatting away about why he loves marathon training.

"I'm proud to be a Clydesdale," he says. Breathless, I nod along with him, but in fact, I have no idea what he means. A Clydesdale? I picture the horses in the old Budweiser commercials, the ones with the fringed hoofs, pulling carts full of kegs. Is he saying he is strong as a horse? That he always pulls his weight in the group?

When I go home and Google the meaning, I discover that Clydesdale is a category in some marathons and other amateur endurance events. It refers to men who are over a certain weight, typically two hundred pounds. I can't find any reference to height, so I deduce (correctly) that Clydesdales are men who are simply heavier, regardless of their height. They can be tall as an NBA player, or short and stout like an Olympic wrestler, or anything in between, so long as they are at least two hundred pounds.

Clydesdales, I learn, also have a female equivalent, Athena. From what I can tell, the Athena category is open to women who weigh 150 pounds or more.

Wait, what?

I read it several times before it sinks in. Slowly, I get up from the computer, go to the bathroom and undress. My bathroom scale is so old it isn't even digital. Only now do I question its accuracy.

My mouth is dry.

Please, don't let me be an Athena.

I pray to Jesus and while I'm at it, Aphrodite, Demeter, Phoebe, and Tethys. There are so many other goddesses I could resemble, instead of Athena, who among her many other accolades, also seems to be the Goddess of Active, Plus-Sized Women.

I take a deep breath, step forward, and hesitate before looking down. When the scale finally settles on a number—144, as I recall—I breathe a sigh of deep relief. Six pounds stand between Athena and me. Thank the Goddess for that.

***

MY JOURNEY TOWARD Boston starts long before I set out to become a runner. It was late January when I first set foot in Boston. I was on my way to Hampshire College, a three and a half hour drive west, in the Pioneer Valley. My covered wagon all packed, I'd been preparing to start in the fall, unaware that my dad hadn't submitted his tax returns to the Financial Aid office as I'd asked. Dad insisted that because he wouldn't be paying for my college anyway, that there was no need for him to do this. But without these documents, my application for financial aid is incomplete. No financial aid, no Hampshire.

To my young adult mind, this sounds like the end of the world. I'm panicked phoning the Bursar's office. A campus administrator told me not to worry; they'd find a workaround. In the meantime, she said, it's better to enter Hampshire in mid-year. That will make the finances smoother. In rural New England in midwinter, it doesn't take long before the walls start to close in. By February, the entire campus will be anticipating the arrival of a few fresh-faced transfer students. The Febutantes, they call us.

I've waited so long to go to Hampshire that I decide I can wait a little longer, and meanwhile, I have a look around Beantown. I check in to a room I reserved in the cheapest reputable-seeming hotel, The Buckminster Hotel in Kenmore Square. I take my first subway ride, to

Cambridge, and meet up with a friend from summer debate camp who is a freshman at Harvard. He sneaks me into the freshman dining hall. The building is decrepit, the food unremarkable. My first taste of privilege, and it's . . . bland? Well, this is a letdown.

But whatever, it's not my final destination. Carefully, I repack my bags, balancing the weight of my belongings for the next leg of my trip, an arduous crosstown journey to the bus station. It is here that I finally board a bus to Hampshire, a forest green coach from a New England-based company called Peter Pan. After barreling three hours through darkness flecked with snowflakes, Peter Pan deposits me, unmagically, on a campus blanketed in snow that has drifted higher than some of the trees.

No one else gets off the bus. My fellow Febs must've already arrived. The coach wheezes and roars away, leaving me in silence. Falling snow sparkles under the amber sodium vapor lamps that barely light the campus, making it look like a New England snow globe come to life. Never again will Hampshire appear this perfect. Smooth and white, it's pristine as a blank page, ripped from my imagination. I drag my rolling suitcase across it, already destroying its perfection.

This is no time to get precious. The academic year is already in full swing. Just to jump in and latch on requires all my focus. Making up for lost time, I sign up for the maximum number of credits allowed, straining the seams of my bookbag with the weight of the reading they require. But I am going to plow through each syllabus, and then some. This education is costing my family and me plenty; I'm determined to get the most from it.

I start out writing for the Hampshire newspaper, but it's so chockablock with satire that it's almost indistinguishable from *The Onion*. I take my earnest journalism off campus, to the weekly in the town of Amherst and later, the *Daily Hampshire Gazette*, in Northampton. For a Hampshire student, this is pretty typical. There is no set curriculum, no majors. Self-directed as we are, Hampshire students tend to identify themselves not by what they study, but what they do.

This makes me a writer, I guess. Later, I'll put a finer point on it. After Hampshire, I enroll in a graduate program in journalism at Stanford University. The program is as much about questioning the conventions of journalism as it is learning to conform to them, so in a sense, it's a like a West Coast version of Hampshire. There is one key difference, though: letter grades. Getting these seems so childish to me, like I'm back in high school.

In addition to taking classes, students are expected to also complete internships in the field. These aren't graded, but it feels like the stakes are still high. I am fortunate to find a paid internship at a business newspaper that covers the rapidly expanding Silicon Valley economy. But it doesn't seem like it'll lead to a full-time job, and I'm not entirely sure I'd take one if offered. My interest in business is not strong enough to overcome the overwhelming downside of a journalism job in the vicinity of Stanford: affordability, or lack thereof.

The fact is, even if I had received perfect letter grades (which I didn't), it would be no guarantee of the A-plus job that everyone in my program seems to be seeking: that elusive entry-level journalism position that pays enough to cover the sky-high Bay Area housing costs, not to mention the car that most of these jobs seem to require.

Instead, I return to Boston newly in possession of a master's degree in journalism, and in what will become a recurring theme, work a temporary administrative job while I figure out what comes next. At least the rent here is much cheaper here than it is in Silicon Valley.

Even though I'm living paycheck to paycheck, I'm fortunate that the abundance of college campuses in Boston means that there are always free events to attend. One evening, I go to MIT to see a documentary about the photographer Cindy Sherman, who is known for taking self-portraits in which she is dressed like other people. At the event, I'm wearing work clothes (meaning: the one suit I own, from Ann Taylor, for job interviews), and as I leave, a man in the audience corners me.

"Cindy?" he says.

He must be joking. Cindy Sherman is decades older than me. Besides, for her to slip into a screening of a documentary about herself would be pretty meta and decidedly weird, even for an artist.

I smile in case he is kidding and tell him I'm not Cindy Sherman. But he doesn't seem to believe me. Here I am in an unknown city, feeling like I'm impersonating a woman with a career and a life, and someone mistakes me for a woman who has made a career and a life out of dressing up as other people.

Leaving the building, I glance back to see the man staring at me intently, as if he's noticed something that everyone else has missed. This makes me feel unnerved, singled out.

And it forces me to consider something. He may be wrong about my identity, but this total stranger has identified a consequential fact of my life: In the entire city of Boston, there is no one who knows who I am.

A warm rush of energy comes over me. This total anonymity is admittedly lonely, but to me, it also feels thrillingly liberating. If nobody knows me, it means I can be anybody.

As I take the T to work in the morning, I see runners on the path along the Charles River. The city is shaping up in anticipation of the Boston Marathon. Banners bearing names of past champions hang from streetlamps. Marathon gear appears in the window of City Sports, a popular athletic store. The long winter is finally waning, and Boston seems ready to bloom. With race day approaching, people from around the world, dressed in colorful running clothing, crowd onto the T. They look excited, and my fellow commuters seem excited for them.

That year, I get caught up in the excitement, too. On the way home from work one balmy evening, I stop into a sporting goods store in the Prudential Center crammed with people buying Marathon gear. I pick out a crisp white running cap with the Boston Marathon logo embroidered in blue. I buy the cap for my brother, Matt, who has just finished his collegiate running career at the University of Portland, hoping that he'll appreciate the running gift. At this point, I don't understand the significance and the import of wearing Boston Marathon apparel.

I'm now pretty sure Matt never wore the cap, not even once. As a serious runner, he knows the unwritten rule that you only wear Boston Marathon items if you've run the race yourself. As a non-runner and newcomer to Boston, I'm oblivious.

But despite my obliviousness that year, the one thing I do know is the location of the marathon's finish line—right in from of the Boston Public Library. Scaffolding and barriers are staged days in advance, impeding me and my fellow bookworms from easy access. Despite this inconvenience, I'm impressed by the scale of the event. It's incredible to behold the city coming together for an international event such as this.

When Marathon Monday finally arrives, it's afternoon before I finally make my way to the finish line. Despite the holiday, I ended up having to work in the morning, and by the time I make it in on the train into downtown Boston, the grandstands are empty. The sky has clouded over, and it's spitting rain. I feel like an idiot, having expected the marathon would still be in full swing so late in the day. All that build-up and I only get to drink in the dregs of the race.

I climb to the top of the cold metal risers anyway and clap whenever someone jogs by. One woman lumbers past, and I cheer fervently for her, but she looks embarrassed and gives me a dismissive wave. She isn't running the Boston Marathon. She is just out for a jog on the still-closed streets.

A few weeks later, I accept a permanent job as a reporter at a newspaper in Panama City, Florida. Before long, the Boston Marathon recedes to the far reaches of my mind, fading to memory by the following year. It is only several years later, as I prepare to run another marathon, across the country in Oregon, that my initial marathon memory washes over me, a friendly wave from a distant shore.

CHAPTER FOUR

The Longest Minute

I THOUGHT THAT, training for a marathon, I'd be running lots of miles. But most of my Portland Fit training plan is written in minutes; only Saturday's long run is assigned in miles. There is no explanation for this seemingly odd training plan. Maybe I'm not yet ready for miles? Are minutes the running equivalent of baby steps? Whoever designed this program must have known I would be looking for a way to speed it up and get it over with.

As I begin training, I realize that minutes have their advantages. I don't need to plot a route, or know how far I've gone, or how fast. I can just head out the door and turn around when half of my minutes have elapsed. What could be simpler? I bet if I opened a copy of *Marathon Training for Dummies,* it would give the same advice.

For two days after the time trial, my legs were sore. But it's not like I never work out. The last time I went to the gym—in the evening so I wouldn't have to pay for parking—I had been unemployed for a little over a week. That was a couple weeks ago. I had joined a nearby 24 Hour Fitness mainly because none of my co-workers were members. I didn't want to spend the day among them, then run into them again while working out at night. A "Gym of One's Own" was what I needed.

But a city as insular as Portland is like the campus of a small liberal arts college, so even stepping out the front door is practically asking to run into someone you know. To see the familiar face of a reporter from a local TV station shouldn't surprise me, but it does. Our eyes meet; there's no way to pretend I haven't seen him.

Ugh, not now. Not him.

In a different context, this guy is actually pretty okay. We became acquainted about a year ago at press conferences and Portland's many political protests. Working for a weekly newspaper, I didn't cover "spot" news like protests, only the issues that precipitated them, but sometimes I went to them anyway. While attending these events, I noticed that, whenever TV news is live on the scene, the protest itself—not the cause behind it—becomes the story.

One rainy evening, I find myself standing on the perimeter of a brick square, chatting with a reporter from a local TV station. We introduce ourselves and lament that a faction of this otherwise peaceful demonstration seems to be getting rowdy. Then, police begin to move in. In minutes, we are engulfed by a sea of people.

I take a few steps back, out of the fray. When I turn around, I catch sight of the TV reporter, mic in hand, getting razzed by the more aggressive members of the black bloc, a loose group of anonymous anarchists known for stirring up mayhem. I felt for him, taking the brunt of collective outrage even as he simply was trying to communicate the point of the collective outrage. It looked like a miserable position to be in. But also, it was a little pathetic.

I ran into TV Reporter a few weeks later, at a Halloween party in a funky old Craftsman-style house in the hippie Hawthorne neighborhood. That's when I softened my stance towards him.

Because it was a Halloween party, all the attendees were dressed in costume. That summer I'd gone to the Pendleton Round-Up, a rodeo in Eastern Oregon, with my mom and aunt. Each of us had come home with cowboy hats, a key ingredient in my cowgirl costume.

TV Reporter was dressed as Joey Ramone, in a cheap, black rocker wig, t-shirt, and jeans. For someone who sometimes fills in as weekend weatherman, it was a self-deprecating choice. Maybe he's not the corporate media stooge I'd taken him for. Maybe that's a costume, too. I should give a little more credit to TV people. The house was crowded and loud; we didn't get the chance to talk. But as I walked out the door, I turned and tipped my cowboy hat to Joey Ramone. He smiled back at me. He knew why I found his get-up so amusing.

Here we are in different costumes: gym clothes. My mind is racing to complete a risk assessment. Does he know I'm no longer at the newspaper? Probably not; I'm no bold-faced name. No one knows or cares. As we slip into idle chitchat, I feel my body relax. A pause comes in the conversation, I know I should fill it immediately, or . . .

"So, what are you doing now?" he asks, suddenly serious.

Too late; he knows. Geez, if I'd wanted to talk about my job, or lack thereof, I would've brought it up by now. Obviously.

"Oh, just some free weights, a little cardio," I say with a smile.

And then, without further ado, I turn on my heel and leave.

In the car on the way home, I cringe at my behavior. He was only trying to be nice. Possibly, he believes I'd been good at my job and, like many before me, had gotten a raw deal. But wasn't it obvious I didn't want to talk about it? Can't a part-time weatherman at least read the current conditions?

Anyway, after that, it's over for me. I call to cancel my gym membership. For most people, a fresh start is joining a gym. My fresh start is quitting one. The woman on the phone informs me I'm paid up through the end of the month and offers to put my membership on hold, indefinitely.

Okay, fine. Hold my 24 Hour Fitness membership for the rest of my natural life.

The gym incident is another reminder of which side I'm on should it ever comes down to flight or fight. Every cell in my body told me to bolt, and I followed this instinct like a wild animal.

What kind of crazy person needs to flee a conversation?

But what's done is done. I'll be better off with Portland Fit, getting outside, out of my head. If there was ever any doubt, this settles it: I'm training for the marathon, starting right this minute.

The plan is to go up residential side streets until it's time to turn around and run back down. Running east, I'll be going away from downtown, away from the gym and its Joey Ramones.

Inspired now, hey, ho, let's go. I click the button on my watch— *beep*—and I'm off. I haven't run these streets before, but I walk them often. Running through then, I'm able to see familiar landmarks in a new light. A couple blocks away on Belmont is Zupan's, a tiny, gourmet grocery with exorbitant prices that I'm always, albeit unsuccessfully, trying to avoid. There's also the Pied Cow, a hippie cafe in a Victorian house with a lovely, decrepit outdoor garden dotted with wrought-iron tables where people choose from a menu of hookah pipes. Someone who used to work there told me about the café's dress code: two slips are the equivalent of a dress, she said, "So, for Portland, it's a bit old-fashioned."

During my run, I stay on the side streets, which are quiet enough that I can run on the smooth, even road, instead of over sidewalks buckled by the roots of trees. It's a cloudy morning, humid, like it wants to rain, but instead, it's probably going to lord it over us all day. The bus roars down Belmont; a garbage truck rumbles in the distance, but somehow, this feels peaceful.

A few blocks and I'm at busy arterial that marks the start of the Laurelhurst neighborhood. I pause to cross the street, but even though I'm just standing, not running, I don't bother to stop my watch. I will not, I decide, be starting and stopping my watch at every intersection. My marathon training minutes are going to be all-inclusive, like Club Med. I look down at my watch.

Wow, it hasn't even been ten minutes yet.

That I even imagined that I could "speed up" my runs to get them over with is now officially ridiculous. Whatever "fast" running is, it is clearly out of the question.

Now that I've made it to the other side of a busy thoroughfare, it feels like a different zip code. Large Craftsman-style homes sit on built-up foundations. Each appears to be inhabited by a single, affluent family, rather than divided into odd-shaped apartments for renters, like the large houses by my apartment.

Rhododendrons and azaleas flourish in these expansive yards; huge bushes bloom early and often. This is the land of Miracle-Gro, or its organic gardening equivalent.

I check my watch; exactly half of my minutes are up. It figures; finally, I've arrived in a place where I wouldn't mind lingering and it's time to turn around.

Back across the busy street, and down Southeast Taylor, a street over from mine. It's downhill all the way, a relief. The blocks go by a little faster, and I return with nearly two minutes to go. Damn. *I could've stayed a little longer up the hill in the nice neighborhood.*

Twenty minutes isn't the same as eighteen, so I make a long loop around the block and approach my door at 19:59 . . . and stop. Click the button. First run done. It's official, I'm training for the Portland Marathon.

When I'd imagined marathon training, I pictured myself tearing through city streets, the background blurry behind me, like the heroine in an action movie. Real-life running, measured in minutes, creeps along slowly, with everything in exquisite focus. I can practically memorize the patterns in the bricks of each apartment building I pass. Never mind "running," I'm barely even moving.

The *opposite* of this is what I'm after. I'd like to speed up my entire life and get to the good part somewhere up ahead. If only I could sprint through surprise encounters with the world's Joey Ramones and their chorus of questions:

So, what are you doing now?
So, what are you doing now?
So, what are you doing now?

I need to get this phrase out of my head.

Next week my schedule bumps me up to thirty minutes, and why not? I've got nothing but time. I trudge up Belmont Street, past the giant hippie sunflower painted in the middle of the intersection. Up ahead, two young men sit on the curb. I can tell from the smell they're sharing a blunt.

I cross to the far side of the street and train my eyes on a crack in the concrete. I'm not moving that much faster than walking. They're going to have plenty of time to get a good long gander at me. As I shuffle by, they chuckle, then erupt into hearty laughter.

Are they laughing at me? Or are they just laughing because they're high? Do I look funny running and sober people are just better at holding back their laughter?

All I know is, nothing like this ever happened at Lloyd Center. One probably shouldn't be shopping when one is not gainfully employed, but if you're young, white, and female in a mall, no one will laugh as you pass them. It's assumed to be your natural habitat.

The streets of Portland, on the other hand, feel like a hostile environment. Out here running, I'm likely to see anybody, or rather, they're likely to see me, wearing shorts.

I'm not Portland Fit, more like Portland Fat. I have no doubt I'll be proud to say I've run a marathon once it's all over; being seen training for one, however, is a different story.

Here's where the cover of darkness comes in. I'm not a morning person, and anyway, it's getting too warm to run past 9 a.m. I will run in the evening after finishing whatever I've set out to do that day. When the light is fading, I'll be less conspicuous. Also, it wouldn't hurt to find deserted areas or unfamiliar neighborhoods in which to log my allotted minutes.

My plan, in other words, is to procrastinate.

One evening it is after dark before I rouse myself from the computer and go outside. It's hard to close the book on all the tasks I need to do: jobs to research, applications to complete, cover letters to write, emails to send using my dial-up internet connection, freelance articles to pitch. Each time I head out, it's getting a little later, but the sun is staying up longer, too. I sit so long sometimes my legs fall asleep.

The yeasty-sweet scent of fresh-baked bread is wafting in the air again. It must be coming from the Franz Bakery down on 11th Avenue. Following my nose like a bloodhound, I run downhill, toward the smell. It leads me, finally, to blocky industrial-looking building painted a pale yellowish white, so that it resembles a giant stick of butter. The aroma of sweet, fresh bread is overwhelming, like a best-selling Yankee Candle scent. I'm nearly halfway through my minutes, but rather than turn on my heel, I make a loop behind the building, hoping to spend a bit more time smelling the glorious carbs. A group of men is standing in a semi-circle. They glance in my direction, uniform in their silence and white coveralls. These are bakers, wearing hairnets, smoking cigarettes. Probably they are wondering what the hell I am doing. That's actually a good question. What the hell am I doing? What am I expecting to find? Even though this a bakery, there is no hearth, no wooden paddle. This is not a bakery in the old world, if such a place ever existed.

The spell is broken as I realize: a commercial bakery is, in fact, a factory that produces bread.

Well, duh.

I knew this, of course. Reality rarely looks as good as it smells, and if I'd bothered to think about it a second, I would probably have saved myself some embarrassment and not come all the way down here.

Oh well, I chuckle to myself as I power back up hill. The smell of bread got me out the door and into my run tonight. I'll take my motivation where I can get it.

A couple of weeks into my Portland Fit training, I call my mom to tell her about my plan to run a marathon. I'm glad to finally have some news to tell, something to suggest progress in a life stuck on pause.

Of course, Mom seems genuinely excited for me, which is nearly always the case; aside from the fact that I'm her daughter, fresh starts are her thing, having reinvented herself several times throughout her own life, including after getting divorced from my dad. Still, even as I hang up, I wish I hadn't told her. I only just started training; maybe I will change my mind about it. Maybe I will get a job and have no time left to run. It wouldn't be the worst thing. With so much up in the air, how can I commit to, of all things, training for a marathon?

If only I could un-dial the phone, reel back my share of the conversation, one word at a time, like the string attached to a tin can. I'm thirty-one years old and still calling my mom to have her be proud of me for something I have barely even begun to do, let alone accomplished.

Having said it out loud, my marathon news seems trivial, a total waste of time. It won't change the world or help the environment, and it sure won't get me the job I need or help repay my student loans or eliminate the de facto student loans known as credit card debt. The marathon is only about me, running 26.2 miles. *Big fucking deal.*

Compounding this fault-finding is the fact that I now can't turn back. No matter how whimsical I may have made it sound, telling my mom about my marathon intentions gives it weight I had not anticipated.

Am I going to run a marathon? Now that Mom believes I am, I've got no choice but to do it. The last person anyone wants to let down is their mom.

CHAPTER FIVE

Running Rebels

In May, Morgan, a friend from Hampshire, invites me to join her in Las Vegas to celebrate her thirtieth birthday. I don't know anyone else who is going, and I don't really feel like meeting new people or partying, but it would be good to see Morgan, and I could use a change of scenery.

Morgan booked a room at the Hard Rock Hotel, and she and Natasha, her friend from LA, make the drive in Natasha's black BMW convertible. It's my first time in Vegas, a place far removed from my Portland bubble.

They pick me up at the airport, top-down on the gleaming Beemer. Morgan offers me a cardboard shoebox full of chocolate chip cookies she baked for the trip. The contrast is classic Morgan: part luxury-loving glamour girl, part eco-conscious do-it-yourselfer (homemade cookies with an upcycled container for them).

Living in LA, Morgan and Natasha are Vegas veterans. As we drive, the two are debating how much to tip and when, as if to one-up each other with knowledge of the etiquette. It sounds like the dark-haired pair intends to grease palms like high-rollers; valet, bellhop, bartender, and concierge all are going to get tipped early and often. I, on the other hand, am spending money I don't really have, so I resign myself to weaker drinks, lesser service, and, whenever possible, carrying my own bags.

But this doesn't bother me, really. Instead, I'm dogged by another thought: Where and when I am going to run?

The hotel charges a separate fee for the use of its trendy gym, and I refuse to pay more good money just to run on a treadmill. The Hard Rock is somewhat off the strip, in an area of the city with long blocks designed for drivers, not pedestrians. Before leaving Portland, I'd looked at a map and noticed that we're not far from the University of Nevada-Las Vegas. For all its car-centeredness, there are sidewalks in the area, and it is not as congested as on the Strip.

After we've settled into our room, I confess to Morgan that there is something I have to do in Vegas. A smile of anticipation lights up Morgan's face, and I realize what I'm about to say will disappoint her. Rather than your typical Sin City excitement—drinking, gambling, getting hitched—I only want to go running. I explain I'm training for a marathon. She asks when it is, and I tell her: October.

Morgan has been applying some mascara to the long lashes that fan out around her large, almond-shaped eyes. They are even wider now, as she turns from the mirror in surprise.

"That's six months away," she says. Morgan pauses, as if doing the mental math, then knowingly nods. Six months: that's about how long it takes a brand-new runner to train for a marathon.

Morgan is cool with my running the marathon, and even my training in Vegas, and I'm relieved to hear it. I appreciate that while it is not something she is into, she can see the appeal. To have revealed my new running regimen to a friend and not been rejected feels like a weight has been lifted.

In the early evening, as Morgan and Natasha relax in the room, I go outside, press the button on my stopwatch, and head toward the UNLV campus. The sun is slanted in the sky, and it's starting to cool off. I can see the lights of the strip beginning to glow. I jog to the end of the block and push the signal for the crosswalk, which seems to take forever to change. I wait, the only pedestrian in sight. Cars whoosh past. Someone rolls down the tinted window of an SUV and yells something unintelligible at me.

When I finally reach UNLV, home of the Running Rebels, I jog laps on the soft grass of the soccer field, eating up time on my digital watch. I make my way back the same way I came, so as not to get lost, although that would be hard to do. The lights of the Strip shimmer in the distance, guiding me like a neon North Star.

At another interminable stoplight, a young man in black pants and a white shirt is waiting, too. He glances at me.

"Hey, you run all the way out here?" he says, which, of course, is stating the obvious.

"I'm training for a marathon," I say, trying my best to sound friendly, not annoyed that he's interrupting my run.

"A marathon?" he says, beaming. The light still hasn't changed; I now fear that it never will.

"How far is that?" He is lit like a casino marquee.

"It's twenty-six miles," I say, omitting the final 385 yards in the hopes of speeding up this conversation.

Close enough, I guess.

"That is a long way," he replies, approvingly. "Damn, that is a long way."

I smile. It's a marathon stoplight. Finally, it turns green. I nod at him in greeting and trot across the intersection.

"Twenty-six miles!" He calls after me gleefully. "That is a loooong way!"

When I get back to the Hard Rock, the giant neon guitar at the entrance is silhouetted by the setting sun. The sky is streaked with my favorite color, pink, and Morgan's favorite color, purple. It's so vivid it's as if switched on by the hotel staff.

I walk into the lobby, past a bar called the Pink Taco, shivering in my shorts and tank top as the air-conditioning blasts my damp skin. I squeeze by people gathered around slot machines, take the elevator up to our plush room. It's Vegas, baby, and while the whole city seems to be pounding drinks, I've been pounding the pavement.

In a way, it's as if I'm a running rebel, too.

CHAPTER SIX

Bookin'

Back in Portland, I run mostly by the digital ticking of minutes. Slowly and inexorably, with my desire for anonymity and my ever-growing volume of training, I cover what seems like every square inch of the wooded city, from the tree-lined streets and stately Martha Stewart colonials of Irvington to the rose gardens and Victorians of Ladd's Addition.

By sightseeing my way through nearby neighborhoods, I have managed to learn how to distract myself from constantly checking my ancient Timex to see how many minutes I have left or try to guess how many steps it will take to burn through them. In this mindset, I'm not a runner; I'm a tourist, a stranger in adjacent lands.

But it's definitely not all flowers and butterflies. I cut through alleys crowded with stinky dumpsters, stretches of busy streets lined with strip malls and gas stations where the sidewalk randomly disappears, not to return for miles.

Much like the graffiti, dog poop, and litter I encounter, boredom soon becomes an inevitable element of running. In fact, I'm now convinced that when you scrape away the sheen of achievement, boredom may form the very foundation of marathon training.

But I know that there are fates far worse than boredom. It's better to be bored doing something than bored doing nothing. Even the most mind-numbing excursion has a purpose. And when I'm done running for the day, I feel satisfaction, a sensation that is otherwise in short supply. Some days it seems the only thing I get right is my run.

Unfortunately, running isn't going to pay the rent. For that, I've acquired, via Craigslist, a temporary, seasonal job involving books. Since I'm a writer who loves to read, this sounds perfect for me. I'm also able to make my own hours, so I'll be able to work around my other freelancing, which is ideal, since I like to be independent.

The pay is surprisingly good, too, but there is one thing about this odd job that lives up to the name. I'm not selling the book or promoting it, at least not in the conventional sense. I'm hired simply to give it away.

When I initially saw the job posting, I feared that the book would be a religious tract, but to my relief, it is a novel, written and published by a wealthy Silicon Valley entrepreneur who, I gather, resents the traditional New York publishing industry and has decided to "disrupt" it.

Already, this effort must have cost him plenty. At first glance, the book doesn't appear self-published. With a beautifully designed hardcover, smooth, heavy pages, and elegant typesetting, it's physically indistinguishable from any mass-market release displayed in giant pyramids at Barnes and Noble.

However, its content marks its difference. As far as I can tell, this novel is awful. The plot is convoluted and off-the-wall. The characters are constructed of cardboard. Heavy-handed spiritual "messages" fall upon the reader like a slap upside the head. A religious tract, now that I think about it, might be easier to digest.

Maybe the book does get better; I'm not about to find out. So bizarre is the prose that, after a few chapters, I stop reading to minimize the lying I'll have to do should anyone ask me about it.

But who am I to judge? The tech entrepreneur-turned-novelist isn't the only one playing make-believe. I figure the job of distributing these books might sound, on my resume, like being a publicist for a small press, a growth industry if there ever was one. The manager who hired me for this job has even encouraged me to cultivate this attitude. But I'm not really promoting or distributing these novels; I'm simply getting rid of them. Although we have never met, the author and I are in cahoots. We've each created works of fiction to further our own agendas.

Working alone, the whole thing feels vaguely covert. The job is physical labor punctuated by a series of logistical challenges. A truck driver delivers pallets of books to a unit I've rented at a nearby storage facility. I rent a van from U-Haul and, equipped with my very own hand truck and box cutters, unload the boxes of books and stack them in the van. Then I drive to festivals, concerts, and other summertime events, passing out hardcovers the way some people hand out CLIF Bars.

It's like a sales job in reverse. On top of a base hourly wage, the more books I give away, the more money I'll make.

There's a catch, of course. In theory, everyone loves free stuff. In practice, it's a lot easier to give people something free to eat, one of life's necessary pleasures, than to get them to take something free to read, which is typically seen as work. Even so, after some time hitting events around the hyper-literate metro Portland area, and with the aid of a few paid helpers I've in turn hired, it is not long before I've begun to saturate the market for *gratis* hardbacks. People pick one up, and when I see them again, at the next brewfest or jazz jam, they have cracked it open and discovered the less-than-profound prose inside.

Eventually, word gets out. Most people simply look away politely when they see me again with my dubious freebie. But every so often someone—usually younger, typically male—will go so far as to call me out, heckling me as I attempt to press another hardcover into the hands of unsuspecting passersby.

"That book sucks!" one shaggy-haired teenage boy hollers behind me one especially humid afternoon.

I try to ignore him and put on my best "Would I lie?" smile as I inform those who ask that it is like a cross between *Into Thin Air* and *Into the Wild*. I know the comparison is off, but I have no idea exactly how inaccurate it is. (Now that I've read both books, I realize I made a ridiculous comparison, and the books I mentioned are by the same author. It was simply the first thing that came to mind. I'd now like to ask Jon Krakauer to forgive me. He did not do a thing to deserve such disrespect; I was desperate to lighten my load and fatten my wallet. We even went to the same college. Jon Krakauer, if you ever read this, I am sorry.)

Miraculously, my pitch appeals to some people, who take the book despite the heckling. Seeing this, others become interested and wander over for a copy, too. Here it is, proof that people are sheep. A steady trickle of passersby trying to get their hands on a book has me emptying boxes of books faster than I can break them down for recycling. After I've given out all the books I've brought, I climb into the van and hightail it back to Portland, praying I'll never see any of these people again.

Giving books away is now officially lucrative, but each dollar is earned by using every muscle in my body. The corrugated metal box that is "my" storage unit is sweltering inside. The ordering, invoicing, stacking, loading, transporting, and scheduling eats up hours. I spend entire weekends and evenings on my increasingly swollen feet, thrusting books into the hands of unsuspecting reader-victims, then searching event calendars for my next battleground. There is also paperwork: orders to be sent in and invoices to be sent out. Now that I have begun to employ helpers, I do their paperwork, too.

Finally, when I've emptied the wooden pallets on which the books are delivered, I must get rid of the pallets to make room in my storage unit for more inventory. This is yet another expense form to fill out, but at least I can do it sitting down.

I also need to stack the pallets in the van and drive them out to a recycling center. The cost of recycling the pallets is determined by weight. An employee instructs me to maneuver the van up a ramp and onto an elevated scale.

Now, this is easier said than done. The scale is high, likely ten, twenty feet off the ground; drive too far and you've gone right off the scale, and it's a long way down. I really don't need to total a U-Haul right now. If only someone else could drive the van up there for me. If only the recycling center had a valet.

Finally, I get the van into place, after being coaxed and cajoled by the scale operator, all the while feeling like a balky horse being forced to stable. Now that I've driven it up here, I'm flummoxed all over again. What about the weight of the van—not to mention me in it?

I ask the scale operator if I should get out of the vehicle. He laughs so hard he practically falls out of his scale operator's shack. I smile and shrug; I'm new to this job. And maybe also, to the concept of subtraction.

The scale operator weighs the van, with me in it, and lowers it back down slowly, like he's being extra-careful not to freak me out. Did he estimate my weight and then deduct it? Maybe I don't want to know. At the window of a nearby trailer, I put the fee on my credit card, without even bothering to note the weight for which I'm paying. Whatever it is, I'll be reimbursed for it.

When I have finally finished stacking books in the scorching metal storage unit and have shuffled through the heat for my assigned number of minutes, I retreat home to my third-floor apartment in an old brick building on Southeast Yamhill Street and lay under the fan I've wedged into the open window.

The city of Portland is shaped in a natural bowl that tends to trap the warm air around downtown. When it's warm, like now, it feels especially thick and heavy. Just to move through it takes excruciating effort. Between the marathon training and my marathon book handing-out, my energy is spent.

I prop my aching legs up against the windowsill. Tiny firings in my quad muscles feel like aftershocks of the day's efforts. The whir of the fan barely drowns out sounds from the street below. A car with no muffler idles outside the Plaid Pantry convenience store.

Summer is settling in over Portland. It looks like I'll be spending it jogging long, slow loops around town and driving in circles around Multnomah County in a van full of books. Neither effort is going to get me anywhere, but at least, when I'm done with them, I'll be too tired to care.

CHAPTER SEVEN
Skinny Happy People

I'M NOT A fast learner. Or at least, this is what a high school teacher once declared, as if such insight sat on a high shelf out of reach and he brought it down for me.

Whether or not it is true, his characterization has stayed with me for all these years. It's unusual for me to do anything—especially physical things—without practicing them first.

Had I known in advance that I would have to run a time trial for Portland Fit, for example, I probably would have time-trialed myself into the ground, and so gotten a pretty accurate idea of what I could expect to run. I would've figured out how to pace myself.

For months now, I've been practicing running. I've faithfully completed my three to four assigned weekday runs and showed up each Saturday for long runs with the green group.

Now a quiz to test my progress: We citizen runners of Portland Fit are assigned to complete a half marathon. Most of the runners in the green group are doing the Helvetia Half Marathon, on June 19. The race is a benchmark on the way to our full marathon in October. Some of my fellow green runners believe the results will help predict our performance in the marathon, but I'm not so sure. October is still four months away.

Thirteen-point-one miles is daunting. But it's all part of the plan, a plan created for beginners like me by someone with much more experience than I. If shorter races aren't on the plan, who am I to contradict it?

Daniel has driven down for the weekend from Seattle and is going to go with me to the race. Although we don't live in the same city, Daniel is my boyfriend, and we're trying out the long distance thing. I know. It's complicated.

We met while we were still undergraduates, years ago in a radio broadcast class—the only class I took at the community college he was attending. Seemingly shy, he had a sense of humor so dry and yet absurd that it was easy to miss if you weren't paying attention. My observant nature was a perfect complement. His witticisms were all the more appealing to me for not being quite so obvious.

Some people just click. We started dating, and when we were together, even the most mundane experience—waiting for a bus, buying a movie ticket—seemed like a fresh adventure. But after only a few months, I was off to Hampshire, and he continued his studies at Washington State University. We talked on the phone and even visited each other's respective campuses, but it's hard to maintain a relationship long distance. I was heartbroken when we broke up, a few months later, a decision that he made, and I had no choice but to go along with it. Although I often wondered whether Daniel and I were destined to be together, I resolved to put such thoughts out of my head. I managed to do this simply by questioning if such a thing was actually even possible, for anybody.

Throughout college, grad school, and post-graduate jobs, Daniel and I would see each other whenever I was visiting my family in Seattle, and it was if no time had passed and nothing had changed.

But at other times I'd hear a faraway, distracted tone of his voice over the phone, and it would confirm for me that the concept of destiny was a myth perpetuated by the patriarchy, or at least, Julia Roberts rom-coms.

I guessed that this was adulthood; we were friends now, a facile word that failed to describe our connection, at least from my point of view.

Daniel's point of view was even harder for me to figure out. I did know that, at least initially, *he* broke up with *me*. So when I'd decided I was moving from Florida to Oregon, and Daniel immediately offered to come down and help me make half of the cross-country drive, I tried to temper my excitement with caution. I didn't want to get my hopes up. Sure, we were setting out on an epic road trip, but on the other hand, hadn't we been down this road before?

Daniel was standing on the curb at the Dallas airport, backpack at his feet, when I drove up to meet him in my overloaded VW. There was barely enough room for his backpack, but we had to make it fit, so we did. We cruised across Texas, over the vibrant red Jemez Mountains of New Mexico and past the Great Salt Lake, staying in cheap motels along the way.

By the time we arrived in the Pacific Northwest, the concept of destiny no longer seemed so crazy to me. Portland was my final destination and his, Seattle, was 200 miles away, but from then on, I knew we would be closer than ever.

Ever since that trip, Daniel and I have beaten a worn path along Interstate 5, traveling back and forth between Seattle and Portland on weekends. Today, he's come down to see me off on my newest endeavor: the half marathon.

While Daniel has never run a half marathon, he is enthusiastic about my doing so. He's generally a fan of all sports, whether spectator or participatory. In high school, he was on the cross-country team, and like me, he also got into long bicycle rides. After college, he started entering bike races.

On one of our first dates, he mentioned having taken part in the Seattle-to-Portland, a well-known local bike ride between the two Northwest cities that can be done in either one or two days.

When I asked which one he'd done, he said the two-day ride: "I'm not an animal."

I smiled; I'd done it in one.

But today Seattle, and even Portland, seem a long way away. The half marathon I'm about to run begins in Hillsboro, near the campus of Intel, the people who came up with the Pentium chip. All I know is there are no real trees in the Silicon Forest. The race begins in an office park.

I prepare my usual pre-run breakfast—plain oatmeal—and put on my race clothes.

We arrive well before the start time. It's a clear, cloudless day, which I fear means it may also be a warm one. The sky is a brilliant blue. Getting out of the car, we enter a stream of smiling runners making their way through the parking lot. The grins on their faces seem perverse, as if they're off to a rock concert, not lining up to run 13.1 miles.

"Look at all these skinny, happy people," I mutter bitterly under my breath. As soon as the words are out of my mouth, I wish I could take them back. It's not what I meant, it's not who I'm trying to be. Bitter, bad Amy has slipped out, and she's as out of place as a punk rock girl at a sorority party.

Seriously, who are these people who are excited to run, an activity I find more punishing than any other physical endeavor? When I played basketball, badly, for one season, in middle school, running was our punishment. If you missed a free throw, you had to run. I ran a lot.

The people all around me are about to cover the equivalent of hundreds of missed free throws and they're going do so of their own volition, likely grinning the whole way. If running is uncomfortable for them, they don't seem to mind. If any of these people are nervous, they show no signs. These must be the optimists of the world, the "can-do" people. Meanwhile I was born to another credo: "What if?"

What if my shoe comes untied? What if I get cramps? What if it hurts? What if I come in dead fucking last?

The staging area is already crowded. I'm astounded so many have shown up so far in advance of the start. I have an excuse for being this early; it's my first race, and I'm nervous. But surely all these others can't also be first-timers? Clearly, half marathoners are not procrastinators like me.

I wonder how they are planning to fill the next ninety minutes until I spot long lines snaking across the sidewalk. Each one winds its way to the front of an aqua-colored Porta Potty. Every few seconds, a door slams open or shut as people move in and out of the turquoise boxes like bees to a beehive.

Luckily, I don't need to go, so I can avoid entering the chaos. This leaves Dan and me with plenty of time to kill, and I'm wondering what we'll do for that long when I notice the head coach of Portland Fit, Paula. Most members of Portland Fit are doing this race as a training run, and for good reason. Paula's race management company runs the event. She and her husband, Dave, are Portland Fit's power couple; the pair coach, run, and own a shoe store where the runners that they train often shop, forming a virtuous circle of fitness and business.

I'm acquainted with Paula since she sometimes runs with the green group, blithely popping Skittles to keep her energy up. Dave isn't in the green group, but he occasionally makes a cameo appearance, joining Paula for part of her run. When she and Dave take walk breaks, they hold hands, a gesture that seems so intimate that I have to look away. This is the first time I have seen Paula in anything other than running gear. She is wearing a short denim miniskirt, and instead of a ponytail, her sun-streaked blonde hair is down and carefully coiffed. It is 8 a.m., and Paula looks ready to party.

I, on the other hand, am wearing baggy black shorts and a black technical tank top from Target; the same thing I wear on every long run. Black may not be the best color choice for such a warm, sunny day, but I hope it is slimming, and I know from experience that it does not become see-through when damp with sweat.

"Hey Paula," I say, and as soon as the words are out of my mouth, it dawns on me that as race director, Paula has got places to be. I don't want to keep her.

But Paula is a pro. Ever so efficiently, she pivots on her heel and flashes her perfect, supermodel smile.

"Heyyyy Amy," Paula exclaims, as if greeting a long-lost friend. "Have a GREAT race!"

I smile back, amused by her effusiveness, disarmed by her apparent sincerity.

Obviously, Paula's happy place is right here, in the staging area for a half marathon she is responsible for organizing.

I wish I shared her enthusiasm. Rather than inspire me, this rah-rah environment is off-putting. I don't want to run with these people; I want to run away from them.

For the next hour, Daniel and I find a rare spot in the shade and wait, chatting a bit, but mostly just observing the first half marathon either us has ever attended. When it's time for the race to start, I give Dan a kiss goodbye. He gives me a cheerful look.

"Have fun."

Fun, really? I may not really know him after all, because now he sounds like Paula, and all the scarily happy people we saw as we arrived. Fun is the last thing that I'd call this.

I strategically make my way toward the back of the pack. Hundreds of runners are crowded together. Not one of them is wearing black. At the bleat of an air horn, runners in front of me surge forward, but no one is running right away. Instead, we wait until those in front begin to slowly move towards the start line.

I and the other runners around me shuffle forward until the crowd thins out, and finally, I am able to break into a jog. Right away I'm regretting my choice to wear black. As I've mentioned no trees in the Silicon Forest, which means there's no shade, but there are other rural markers, like grass and cows.

From the start, I'm breathing hard, inhaling the smell of cow dung with every breath. *It's gonna be a long race.*

But somehow my training kicks in, and I'm able to make it through the first two-thirds of the race. At mile ten, I tell myself I'm in the home stretch, but my stomach is cramping badly. I feel the urge to use the bathroom, but I don't see any portable toilets, and anyway, the thought of stopping to use one is entirely unappealing.

Cue the wave of panic; each footfall jostles my stomach even as it brings me closer to the finish line and a much-needed bathroom.

I try to distract myself from what my gut is saying. I focus on the runners in front of me. I look at the golden grasses and weeds, the rolling not-quite-farm country around me.

I know I can wait; I must wait.

Long gone is the smell of cow dung, which helps. I'll be there soon, as long as I keep moving forward. I concentrate on taking a single step at a time.

Eventually, a blue finish line banner comes into sight. I want to go faster to finish sooner, but I fear that increasing my exertion will upset the delicate détente I've made with my gut.

No, not yet. Hold on.

I lumber past the giant, white race clock and at long last over the rubber mats that record my chip time, officially 2 hours and 25 seconds. Someone loops a finisher's medal around my neck, but I barely pause as I slow to a walk. I have another finish line in mind. I race-hobble to a cement structure that houses the park's bathroom.

As I enter, I breathe a sigh of relief, but I'm surprised to find I can't go.

I have been holding it for so long, how is this possible?

In the dark stall, I slow my breath and try to relax. I did it, I can let go now.

Things eventually and thankfully return to normal, which makes me happier than I've been all day, almost as happy as the runners I saw as we arrived. To have finished a half marathon is one thing; what I'm truly grateful for is to have finished without having an accident. I walk a bit and find Dan in the finish area, waiting for me, with my friend Kristy, who must've arrived after the start.

Kristy has run a half marathon. She has felt the same pride, the same discomfort—well, most of it anyway. When I tell Kristy my finishing time, she says it's around the same time as her first half marathon.

Yay! I am normal.

Now that all this is settled, I'm suddenly, inexplicably hungry.

There is a post-race barbeque, so I wait in line to collect a charred veggie burger slapped onto a soft, white hamburger bun. I slather it with mustard and ketchup to make edible what I expect to be a mighty bland offering. But from the first bite, I'm amazed at the vibrant flavor of the sweet, tomato-y ketchup and the salty, savory soy patty. So good. I offer Kristy and Daniel some of my food. "Really, it's good," I say, but they decline, just as normally, I would, too.

How can this Costco picnic food suddenly taste so delicious? Oh, yeah. Maybe it's because I just exercised for over two hours.

I enjoy every bite, clean my plate, and toss it into the trash. Kristy and I make plans to meet up again. At the car, Dan and I quickly unload cardboard boxes. As runners pass us on their way to their vehicles, we hold out books for them to take. People accept them happily, and nobody seems to recognize me, or the book in my hand. In minutes, all the books we've brought are gone.

Never have I given away a car full of books so quickly. It's a book distribution personal record. For the first time in a while, I'm satisfied.

We drive home with a car full of empty boxes, proof I really have left it all on the course.

CHAPTER EIGHT
Home Is Where You Make It

IT'S THE LATE 1970s, and I'm in elementary school, eager for summer to start. Mom says the murky, bottle-green waters of Lake Sammamish are off-limits until the thermometer outside the back door reads 70 degrees Fahrenheit. The moment the mercury cooperates, my older sister, Melissa, and I will head down the hill with our towels, wade out to the mossy dock, and jump off, shrieking as cold water shocks our warm bodies. Laughing, shivering, we'll hurry out, towel off, and do it again.

But summer always ends, and this one is no different. Dad moves out, taking with him cardboard boxes of barware for his tavern in Seattle, which has been like a second home for him for as long as I can remember. It's a time of turmoil in my little corner of the world. He and my mom are about to divorce.

Meanwhile, on the other side of the globe, a revolution is taking place in Iran. I know this from TV and because, when Mom decides to have a moving sale, a friendly family with three children roughly the same ages as me, Melissa, and my brother, Matt, show up to peruse our offerings. They have just escaped Iran with little more than the clothes on their backs and so are in need of furniture. Perfect timing, 'cause we've got to get rid of ours.

The Iranian mom and dad haggle good-naturedly with us over the chairs and sofa we've arranged on the driveway as if it's a stage on *The Price is Right*. Hamming it up in front of our friendly new acquaintances, Matt attempts to sweeten the deal by throwing in a brass table lamp.

"Package deal," he says, and everyone laughs.

What they don't buy goes with us—Mom, Melissa, Matt, and I—to a two-bedroom apartment behind a Safeway supermarket far from any body of water, natural or man-made. Six months later we have to move again, to a bigger apartment in a sprawling suburban complex called Kings Place, which had an outdoor pool.

Melissa, now a high-schooler, spends her summers babysitting, while Matt, two grades below me, spends them on the basketball court. I spend the summer before sixth grade in the pool. I can see it, glowing at night, from the window of the bedroom Melissa and I share. It's like the pool is calling to me, a respite from boredom and drudgery.

The neighbor kids and I take turns seeing who can swim farthest underwater before coming up for air. I make it my summer's goal to conquer these competitions. I can swim to the wall and back and half-way back again, nearly three lengths. I relax, conserve my oxygen, and take as few strokes as possible, gliding the momentum out of each one. Once I've mastered this, no can beat me at it.

Unfortunately, I never swim nearly as well at high school swim meets where swimming well matters. There are two kinds of high school swimmers; girls who grew up swimming year-round on age-group teams, and swimmers—like me—just starting to compete.

In seventh grade, I'd attempted to start my official swimming career as a member of the local club team, the Dolphins. However, it required too much (which is to say, any) fundraising and someone to drive me to practice. So, when the activities bus roars up to my junior high, I'm first in line, ready to start all over again.

The high school swim team takes all comers who have achieved the ripe old age of ninth grade. Participants get team suits, team photos, team everything. All of it is royal blue (for we are the Royals, especially those of us from Kings Place) and none of it is free. But when summer comes, I take a lifeguard training class and immediately get hired as a lifeguard and swim instructor at the public pool on my high school's campus. I'm grateful my ability to swim has enabled me to quit my current part-time job at Domino's Pizza. In more ways than one, swimming is finally starting to pay off.

The pools where the team swims are all indoors, windowless worlds unto themselves. In the middle of a lifeguarding shift or a team practice, it's hard to tell whether it's day or night, summer or winter. Tiny lights shine from the ceiling like stars. In the water, I'm weightless and untethered, an astronaut in outer space.

My senior year, the pool is still closed for maintenance when fall practice is supposed to start, so instead, we do our workouts at a private swim club. An outdoor lap pool is something I've only heard of before. Now I am immersed in one, with the blue sky above, green trees all around, black line steady beneath me. For two weeks we swim laps in the late summer sun, giddy at the tan lines we are getting. It's awesome, the perfect note on which to end my time in competitive swimming.

There is no swim team at Hampshire College, which is fine by me. After years enduring a sports-trumps-everything environment, I'm happy to train my mind, not my body.

For so long I felt starved for academic choice. Now I'm overwhelmed with options. Because Hampshire is part of a college consortium, its students can choose from classes at four other schools. Every course in the catalog sounds fascinating; I want to sign up for all of them.

Hampshire students create their own majors. The one I'm designing includes all kinds of subjects: film, television, history, law, and a kind of newish discipline called critical theory. I'm not sure exactly how to define it—it seems like a sort of philosophy—but nonetheless, I find it fascinating. The academics immersed in it seem to constantly be coming up with influential ideas and then conveying and debating them at conferences and in the pages of journals and magazines.

How all of this adds up to gainful employment is beyond me. Critical theory is cool, but I know that soon this fake adulthood will be over, and I will have to find a way to repay the loans I've taken out to be here. Certainly, I won't be able to do this by lifeguarding.

To that end, I focus not only critiquing media but learning how to make it. I really don't see how you can do one well without also doing the other, but some of my professors keep telling me that sooner or later, I'll have to choose.

They may be right. As graduation approaches, I'm unsure how to keep going on the mishmash of subjects I've been studying. A PhD in communications or American studies? Some sort of fellowship? The path before me is obscure.

Journalism, on the other hand, is tangible, intuitive—just tell the stories that need to be told, and don't overthink them. I decide to earn a master's degree in journalism at Stanford University, because as I understand it, the program's philosophy is that there should be no false distinctions between media theory and media-making. They're interrelated, interdependent. Sign me up; this is exactly what I've been saying all along.

The main entrance to Stanford University's campus, Palm Drive, is like something out of the opening credits of *Beverly Hills, 90210*. True to its name, towering palm trees line the boulevard, which leads to an oval filled with flowers in the university's colors, cardinal red and white. Sand-colored buildings with red-tiled roofs stand grandly around it, like palaces of a Renaissance city-state. Visually, it's stunning, albeit a little grandiose.

But for me, Stanford's biggest reveal is its pool. An emerald-cut sapphire that sparkles in the year-round sun, the pool is, in fact, four outdoor pools set together as one. When I learned I'd been awarded a fellowship to earn a master's degree, it never occurred to me that access to extravagance would be included. It will be weeks before I get up the gumption to return with my suit and goggles. Janet Evans, Summer Sanders, and other Olympic medalists have trained in these lanes. Those are some pretty big strokes to follow.

Posted on the locker room walls are signs for lessons like the ones I used to teach. And at the far end, a PhD student from my department is backstroking slowly in a swim cap covered with rubber flowers. Looking around, I know that I'm more than qualified to swim here. All it takes is a student ID.

As for my studies, the program is small and intense; filled with Type-A people who appear determined to achieve big things. And we are pretty much outnumbered by those around us who have already made their mark. Accomplished mid-career journalists are here at Stanford for a year-long fellowship and look, for the most part, as if they never want to leave.

Because I was not a journalism major at Hampshire, I start out already behind and must make up some required credits in technical skills, like copyediting. The curriculum requires so much focus that by the time I pull my head up from my thesis and internship and have a look around, final exams are over. I feel as if I've hardly gotten here and already it's time to leave for the real world. I've decided that for me this means print journalism.

As so many experienced journalists remind me, it's a risky decision. The newspaper industry is in free-fall nationwide, but Florida, America's third most populous state, features a churning newspaper market with an ever-present need for new (read: cheap) reporters.

Also, it's sunny there. I'm in.

I eventually take a job as a reporter at a daily newspaper in Panama City, in Northwest Florida, which is also known as LA, short for "Lower Alabama."

Panama City's claim to fame—and it's biggest industry by far—is Spring Break. Each year, starting in March, college students from around the country flock to the emerald waters and white-sand beaches of Panama City Beach. The rest of the year, it lives up, or down, to its other nickname, the Redneck Riviera.

Panama City is a relatively recent destination for Breakers. Once upon a time, Fort Lauderdale used to be the big draw. That was before business leaders, wanting to make the city more upscale, made it clear hard-partying college students were no longer welcome.

So there is a satisfying symmetry when, after a couple years as a reporter in Panama City, I pack up and head south, to Fort Lauderdale, and a job writing for an alternative weekly. The city formerly known as Fort Liquordale and I are both trying to move up in the world.

Residents of the city insist the safest, cleanest, and overall nicest places to live in Fort Lauderdale are found between the highway and the beach, a densely-populated strip of real estate with hit-and-miss affordability. Wanting to live in the most central location possible, I've leased the cheapest apartment within it, a one-bedroom just inside the rainbow flag boundary of the Fort Lauderdale's oldest gay neighborhood, Victoria Park.

A couple of miles away from my apartment are not one but *two* Olympic-size outdoor swimming pools, both open to the public year-round. Lap swim only costs a few bucks.

It's an opportunity that's too good to pass up. But it's been years since I swam laps with any regularity; my flip turns are awkward, water goes up my nose. Yet the scent of chlorine is like perfume to me, evoking carefree afternoons at Kings Place, with my lane-mates on the swim team, at Hampshire College during undergrad, and most recently at Stanford University. Now I can add South Florida to the list.

I start to swim regularly in the evenings, after work. As I lift my arm to breathe, I can see the sunset sky reddening, triangular backstroke flags flapping in the breeze. The white globe lights around the pool are on, shining like an early moon. Fort Lauderdale is far from the moneyed perfection of Palo Alto, but its pools and palm trees give it a touch of Stanford glamour. Already I can tell that Fort Lauderdale will be a hard place to have to leave.

At a session at the pool, I learn about an upcoming sprint triathlon: swim, bike, run. Unlike the triathlons I've seen on television, it requires no wetsuit, no road bike. It's about as entry-level as triathlon gets. I'm game.

The half-mile swim takes place in Miami's Biscayne Bay. Unlike the ocean, the bay is protected, sandy-bottomed, and clear enough for snorkeling. Compared to the cold, choppy waters of Lake Washington, where I'd competed in mile-long open water races during my high school swimming days, a swim in the bay should be no problem.

The bike portion of the race is a ten-mile loop on a flat, paved course. Growing up, I often rode my bike farther than my mom allowed, determined to discover whatever lay just on the other side of the seemingly arbitrary boundary she set. Mom noticed my enthusiasm for cycling and when I was in junior high, bought me a twelve-speed racing bike for my birthday, entry-level by serious cyclist standards, but lighter and faster than anything other kids owned. By high school, I was competing in organized bike rides throughout the region, covering up to two hundred miles in one day. So ten miles should be no problem.

But in college and grad school, and since then, I have cycled only sporadically, mostly just as a way of getting from Point A to Point B. My current bike reflects my haphazard approach. It is a mountain bike I bought at a pawn shop, pawn shops being the default bike shops around here. South Florida roads and drivers are so unfriendly to cyclists that few people seem to bother with road bikes. The race organizers must recognize this; the race has a division just for people riding mountain bikes and other upright bikes, which are much slower than racing bikes, with their sleek frames and skinny tires. Ten miles upright on a knobby-tired mountain bike would be pokey but comfortable, totally doable.

So while the swim and the bike thirds are pretty much covered, it's the run section that intimidates me. A 5K (3.1 miles) run is farther than I've ever gone on foot. It's so hot down here, and it's not even summer yet. I'm convinced that I'd faint if I tried to run outdoors. The only place I see people running is on a soccer field, or on treadmills in air-conditioned gyms.

I've never really been much of a runner—I've only shuffled a couple miles along suburban sidewalks mostly for something to do, or as a way to get in shape for swimming.

But I'm determined to try my best to train for this triathlon. I do all the running required to prepare by making multiple rounds on the dirt path that winds through Holiday Park, a green buffer between downtown and the residential area where I live.

Homeless people often lug their bags through the park, and in the late afternoon, people still in their work uniforms sometimes come here to walk the mile-long loop.

One day I jog past a couple of people walking on the dirt path.

"Walking burns more fat," one of them calls after me.

Walking burns more fat. As if the *sine qua non* of physical activity is to incinerate adipose tissue. I don't take it personally. She's probably a personal trainer, speaking for the benefit of her client, whose efforts she is paid to affirm. After all, in South Florida, fat-elimination is big business. Ads for "fat-burning" herbal supplements are everywhere you look. Billboards advertise plastic surgeons trained to "sculpt" the body. If jumping off a causeway burned fat, South Florida's fitness "professionals" would probably offer classes in it. It seems like I'm one of the few residents exercising for a non-fat-burning reason.

Soon, repeated loops of Holiday Park are getting boring, and the place is off limits after dark for safety reasons. But I have an idea. One evening I head past the boutiques and rococo condos of Las Olas Avenue, turn down a creepy underpass, and head along Federal Highway to enter the quiet confines of a planned community called Rio Vista.

I first discovered this neighborhood on a boat tour of Fort Lauderdale's canals and waterways, which are the reason the city calls itself the Venice of America.

On the tour, boat passengers *ooh*ed and *ahh*ed at the waterfront homes lining the Tarpon River. For people living in them, the river was practically a backyard. Most homes had expansive tiled terraces open right out onto it, the better to see and be seen by passing yacht traffic. Some people, sunning themselves by their pools or puttering about their gardens, waved at the folks on the boat. As I begin to look for alternate running routes, I realize how beautiful a path that this would be.

Unlike other affluent Broward County neighborhoods, this one isn't gated. There is no checkpoint at the entrance. Open to all and yet peaceful as can be, Rio Vista, a real estate agent might say, is an oasis in the heart of the city.

Revived by the sight of its gold and stucco sign, I jog down the street, but it's less idyllic than I remembered. Oh well. I should've realized there'd be no vista of the Rio. Mediterranean villas are mostly hidden behind massive walls, covered in bougainvillea, impassive as fortresses. Like a well-designed resort, it's hard to see which way the road will turn, making it seem like I'm perpetually on the verge of discovery.

This neighborhood was first built shortly after World War II, but it is obvious some of the original homes were razed to make way for grander versions of the same. Like men's summer shirts in a catalog, they are arrayed in complementary shades of mustard, ochre, and terra cotta.

I make my way through the labyrinth of villas, wondering what life is like inside them. Fronds of palm trees rustle in the breeze. The landscaping is lush, fragrant with the scent of white flowers opening at night. It smells like a bike ride home to my apartment in Palo Alto.

It is hard to believe I'm still in Fort Lauderdale, with its abundance of 7-Elevens and tire stores, "a tropical paradise," as the art director at work likes to say, with a sardonic smile.

So many people have staked a claim on the south end of this thin strip of land that it is rare to find a place to yourself. However, many of these houses must be unoccupied, as they are more than likely used as second homes of the wealthy. They sit empty while their owners are somewhere else, amassing the fortune required to afford them. And now I enjoy their solitude, for free.

It's hot at night, and I'm still not used to it. South Florida swelters around the clock. My jog has slowed to a shuffle that soon becomes a glorified walk.

Maybe it's time to head back. One of these streets has got to connect to the highway.

The street dead ends. I try another, but it's a cul-de-sac. I'd turn around, but I can't seem to remember which way I came. Hidden somewhere among the palm fronds, security cameras are probably filming me. If anyone is monitoring them, I must look ridiculous. I hope no one ever sees the images of me increasingly becoming desperate to get the fuck out of Rio Vista.

I'm practically walking now. But walking burns more fat!

It must be so cool inside those homes, if there is even anyone there. Maybe someone will get a pizza delivered, and I can ask the driver for directions. I'm surprised there's no private security guards patrolling in faux squad cars.

I've got to be close to getting out. It's a little late at night to go around knocking on doors, asking for directions. And mostly there are no doors; just wrought iron gates with intercoms mounted on them. So I keep moving.

My hips ache. I've got to keep going. They say you can drown in as little as six inches of water. It's also possible to lose one's mind and all sense of place in a neighborhood with numbered streets. Wait: numbered streets. What street was on I when I entered this place? No idea. Maybe just try to go to the lowest number? How long has it taken me to realize this?

I work my way back, 18th Street, 17th, 16th . . . Homes I swear I didn't pass now appear before me.

Have I run this street? Am I going back the way I came?

I stop and listen for the siren song of South Florida: traffic from a nearby highway. All I hear is the hum of an air conditioner. It's demoralizing.

Okay, just a second of rest.

I suck in my breath and look up, letting all of it out. There are no stars in South Florida. To refer to the night sky as heavens seems profane, polluted as it by artificial light. But wait. I can see the glare from businesses on Federal Highway. Blockbuster Video's fluorescent sign is throwing blue and yellow beams like an undiscovered planet.

Light pollution: my salvation. Beam me up, Scotty.

I run toward the light, and finally, I reach the same entrance I came in, pass the Rio Vista sign, and return to the real world. It's just a straight shot to my apartment now, sidewalk all the way. Finally, back in familiar surroundings, I start picking up speed.

Flat and freckled with strip malls, Fort Lauderdale is an ordinary place transformed by the slanting sun. Daybreak and sunset are her most flattering angles. After dark, not so much.

Cars whoosh by on Federal Highway, and I keep my head down, avoiding headlights. You don't want to look up, as a pedestrian on Federal Highway at night. You don't want to give anyone driving by a reason to stop and offer you a ride.

I am famished when I get home and yet too tired to do more than pour cereal into a bowl. It's so good to be home, in my tiny, tidy, concrete-block apartment. The cereal tastes amazing. I fall into bed, sticky with sweat. I'll shower it off in the morning.

Only a moment seems to have passed when the fierce Florida sun blazes through the spaces between my blinds. My knees ache, my head aches, strangely, my hips hurt, too. It's like a full-body hangover, but I haven't been drinking.

Go away, sun!

Suddenly I remember, last night, the epic run. I get out of bed, pull up a map on my computer and, with the same anticipation I feel when checking the newspaper for my byline, try to determine the distance I covered. If you drive a straight line—which, obviously, I didn't—it is about two and a half miles from my apartment to the entrance of Rio Vista, so that's five miles round trip, not counting how far I went wandering around, then trying to find a way out.

Seven miles I covered last night? Eight?

I'll never know for sure exactly how far I ran; Rio Vista keeps her secrets. Certainly, it's farther than I've ever gone on foot.

It was terrible. I was exhausted, confused. But also, incredible: I was running for nearly two hours! I ran seven or maybe even eight miles.

I shut my laptop.

Now there's no need to worry about a 5K. I'll make it.

CHAPTER NINE

Long Runs Are My Louis Vuitton

EVERYONE HAS A unique relationship with time. Some of us live for today, some dwell in the past, and others' minds are focused on the future. I am a future-focused person, and right now, it's a burden. Being unemployed and looking for a job is especially nerve-wracking for me and my fellow future-focused people, who think a lot about what is about to happen and worry about how best to influence it.

Luckily, having a goal of running the Portland Marathon in October and a plan for how to achieve it alleviates some of this stress, because completing this race is at least one positive thing I can count on happening.

In the future, I will learn the reasons for this. In 2010, I read *The Time Paradox* (2008) by psychologists John Boyd and Philip Zimbardo, which describes how each person has a specific orientation towards time. One tendency that the book identifies is "present hedonism," meaning the tendency to savor sensual pleasures in the moment.

We all know at least one hedonist. That person never fails to appreciate when a meal is delicious or when a sunrise is beautiful. Because they are always responding extra-fervently to whatever they are presently experiencing, hedonists can be a little annoying. At times it's as if their default mode is permanently stuck on "ecstatic." Moaning with pleasure at every sip of wine, shrieking at the beauty of a snowfall when everyone else is freezing, hedonists seem starved for attention. But, if you can get past the constant, cringe-inducing *mmm*-ing, their sincere zest for life can be contagious.

A self-assessment in the book indicates that I am a present hedonist about 20 percent of the time. Training for the Portland Marathon, my hedonistic side must be on sabbatical, because for me to enjoy anything feels effortful, unnatural, and almost impossible.

I cannot imagine how running—sweaty, awkward, boring running—could ever bring me pleasure while I'm doing it. But what I come to discover is that long runs warp one's perception of time, either speeding it up so that it passes in the blink of an eye, or slowing it so grossly that passing through fifteen miles feels equivalent to living through fifteen years.

Every week, the green group meets near the Willamette River and runs mostly along paved bike paths and over bridges, going a little farther on each outing. I simply try to keep up the pace and my end of the conversation, letting more experienced runners keep track of time and distance.

On runs like these, time seems to be slowing down. The longer a run lasts, the more pronounced this effect. The last thirty minutes of a fourteen-mile run stretch out before me like a hunk of saltwater taffy.

On the occasions when I can't make the Saturday group run, the prospect of doing a long run alone makes me anxious. The training schedule sets the objective and it's always incremental, but there's no telling what it will feel like, and it is usually more intolerable when I'm alone, with no one to distract me. This is why, even though I lay out my clothes the night before, when running alone I still change them several times. No single outfit seems appropriate for all the elements and microclimates I might encounter during an hours-long run. It's such a long time to be out there all alone! With only the clothes on my back—they'd better be exactly the right clothes.

Before heading off on the first of my solo runs, I check a map and wonder: *How many squares on this grid will I cover? Where are the hills, and can I avoid them?* For the fuel that I'll need at some point, I pour watermelon Gatorade into a bottle and dilute it to a very specific ratio, as more experienced runners have instructed, and tuck a plastic sandwich bag of gummy bears in my pocket.

Rituals of preparation now complete, I step outside, hit the timer on my watch, and set off on the mean streets of Portland. I have no way of gauging distance. I am supposed to cover ninety minutes out, and ninety minutes back, and basically just keep running, no matter how slowly I wind up moving. Other than that, there are no rules. Each turn, each decision, is entirely up to me. I'm on a journey into the unknown: I can run down a street I've never been before just to satisfy my curiosity.

This freedom is appealing. With a whole city to discover, it feels like the world is my oyster! Fast-forward an hour or two, and the bloom is off Rose City. Turns I've spontaneously decided to take have led me up and over steep hills, killing my legs and nixing any desire to explore. I've blown through my bag of gummy bears, drained the Gatorade, and refilled my bottle with the metallic-tasting swill from a water fountain.

Things turn even more ominous as the sky clouds over. Dark thoughts roll in: *I am no good at running; I don't look like a runner. I don't know where I am going, both on this run and in life. How much money do I have in my bank account, and how much do I owe on my student loans? Will I ever get a real job again?*

Hours of swinging them at my sides have made my arms feel rusted out by the Portland rain. My legs ache from pounding them against the pavement; I'm pretty sure they're forming premature varicose veins. The soft tissue around my knees crackles as if Pop Rocks are embedded in my skin.

I want to be done right now. I do not want to run another step. But I've got at least thirty minutes of running left and no car, no cash, and no phone. My legs are my only way home. I'm forced to continue. When I finally get home in one piece, it will feel like I've accomplished a monumental feat.

Repeated exposure to the tedium of long runs makes me think of them as the Chinese finger traps my siblings and I used to play with as kids; the more you struggle, the more the trap constricts. On an hours-long run, obsessing over how much time is left and wishing it would elapse faster only make things worse. Yet that is exactly what I'm doing—constantly glancing at the digital countdown on my wrist to see how many minutes before I can turn around and make my way back.

It's no use. Runs lasting several hours are mandatory for marathoners, especially those training for the first time. Looking ahead at the training plan, I see that I will have to do runs of up to twenty miles. Running this way, so impatiently, is not making anything easier, so I devise a plan. I will force myself to pay extra attention to everything around me. All the houses I see, every bird or tree, I'm going to observe these as if seeing them for the first time. As if there's going to be a pop quiz at the end, I will at least try to memorize every mile.

Once, in the pages of *Runner's World*, an actress described her long, slow runs as "luxurious." First reading it, her choice of words seemed incongruous, if not downright ridiculous, to me. This is a woman who owns Christian Louboutin stilettos. How could she put long, slow runs in the same category?

Even for those who have access to luxury goods, there is, I have begun to recognize, yet another level of extravagance. Time is the only thing you cannot acquire more of, which makes it the ultimate limited edition. To spend time on an activity with a value that is only intrinsic is to experience what sociologists call leisure luxury.

Leisure luxury. I hadn't thought of marathon training as a leisure activity, since for me it feels like work, a project in self-improvement. But because I am never going to get paid for it, running must be the opposite of work: leisure. And certainly, I take my time while doing it.

Whenever I manage to immerse myself in my surroundings, running becomes a different experience. Slowly, leisurely covering what seems like every square inch of the wooded city, I marvel at all that I've missed. Winding through nearby Forest Park and up to the reservoir at Mt. Tabor, I jog tree-lined boulevards, cross bridges made of steel and painted brick red or pale green, shuffle along the turgid brown Willamette River, and make my way over floating docks connected by creaky aluminum footpaths. I take detours off the city's wider main drags—Glisan, Morrison, Stark—and into undiscovered neighborhoods just to take a look at their colorful bungalows, sunflowers towering in immaculate backyards.

Though I've never heard anyone use the term leisure luxury in an actual conversation, I am beginning to appreciate its essence. Even though I dread it beforehand, and also though it leaves me utterly depleted at the end, by concentrating on all this around me, my long runs now feel like something I *get* to do, rather than something I *have* to do. To lavish hours on the most unremunerated activity—running slowly—is something few can afford. It's not a burden but a privilege. Time spent on long runs has indeed come to feel more precious than a

Rolex, more indulgent than Carrie Bradshaw's infamous collection of Manolo Blahniks.

I do a little reading, and it turns out I am on to something in experiencing running as a luxury. Studies have shown increased participation in endurance sports tends to make people less materialistic. As far as I can tell, the reasons for this have not been established. Maybe people come to crave endorphins because they last longer than the brief mood spike of "retail therapy." Or maybe all this physical exertion just makes people too tired for places like Lloyd Center.

Whatever the case, I don't need to read more research. I am a data point of one, and long runs are my Louis Vuitton.

CHAPTER TEN

No Girls Allowed

On the weekend, doing laundry in the basement of my apartment, I run into the apartment manager, Rosie, whose father owns the building. She asks what I'm up to, and I mention that I'm training to run the Portland Marathon in October.

Rosie seems unimpressed. "The marathon?" she says drily. "Well, don't have a heart attack."

I know Rosie is joking. She's actually referring to a mythical run by a Greek soldier tasked with bringing the news of Greece's victory over Persia to Athens from the plains of Marathon, where the decisive Battle of Marathon was fought, in 490 BCE. The runner, believed to be Pheidippides, is said to have delivered his message, "Rejoice, we conquer," and died on the spot.

Death: the ultimate punchline.

Rosie's joke isn't that funny to me, but at least she knows her history. A little more background: the first modern Olympic Games, held in 1896 in Athens, were a revival of the legendary competitions in ancient Greece, so of course they included a recreation of the mythical run from Marathon to Athens, a distance of 24.5 miles. And the winner of that first "official" marathon race was a Greek runner, Spyridon Louis, who, at twenty-three years old, arrived at the finish line in Athens 2 hours, 58 minutes, and 50 seconds after he started, and he didn't have a heart attack or die on the spot. He lived to be sixty-seven.

Some men who saw the race were inspired and brought the idea back to America. The next year, the first Boston Marathon took place on

April 19, 1897. Fifteen men entered. Called the American Marathon, it started in Ashland, Massachusetts, and rambled 24.5 miles to Boston's Copley Square.

No women entered. The event would for decades be held as a men-only event, just like the modern Olympic marathon on which it was modeled, and the ancient Greek games before that.

It took a couple determined women to change things.

Bobbi Gibb grew up in the Boston suburbs, and a friend of her dad told her about the Boston Marathon. (By this time, both the start and finish of the race had been moved; the marathon covered the now standard 26.2 miles.) Bobbi went out to see it in 1964 and was captivated. The next day, she started her training.

In the 1960s, regular people weren't into running. Neither men nor women went "jogging" for the fun of it. The mainstream running boom was nearly two decades away.

But for women, running wasn't just strange, it was also taboo. It was then a popular belief that women's bodies couldn't withstand the strain of running so far. It was nothing personal; just the facts. Some even went so far as to say that a woman's uterus would fall out if she stressed herself so much. In other words, she'd become less of a woman.

Bobbi Gibb had heard all of this, and she questioned its validity. In February 1966, she wrote a letter to the Boston Marathon race organizers, asking for an application. She got a letter back, saying women weren't allowed because they weren't physiologically capable of completing a marathon.

Physiologically capable? That was the problem? Bobbi had a solution. She'd disprove it.

Bobbi's parents were worried when she told them of her plan to "bandit" the Boston Marathon. But when she explained why, her mom understood the reasoning behind it. (Shout out to Bobbi Gibb's mom.) She drove Bobbi to the start line in Hopkinton. Bobbi waited in the bushes. After the start, she jumped into the pack. She'd worried she'd be thrown out when others noticed a girl in the midst, but the runners around her were supportive, and spectators cheered her on.

Bobbi Gibb finished the race in 3 hours and 21 minutes, in a black tank swimsuit and rolled up Bermuda shorts, looking, to my 1990s eye, like a model in a J.Crew catalog. When she crossed the line, the governor was there to shake her hand. A newspaper headline declared her the first "gal" to run the marathon. She was twenty-three.

You'd think that Bobbi finishing in the middle of the pack of men would show race organizers that females running a marathon were no danger to themselves, or anyone else, and cause them to change their now-disproven rules, and let "gals" in.

Well, that didn't happen, but Bobbi's run was the start of something.

The same year, in upstate New York, Kathrine Switzer was studying journalism at Syracuse University and training with the men's cross-country team, since there was no team for women.

As they ran together in the sleet and snow, Kathrine's coach, Arnie Briggs, regaled her with stories of the Boston Marathon. Eventually, Kathrine had enough of hearing about it, and she suggested they just run the race.

But women weren't allowed, Arnie said.

Bobbi Gibb, Kathrine countered. Bobbi did it.

Arnie said he'd take her to Boston if she could prove she could do it by running the distance in practice first. Three weeks before the race date, they ran twenty-six miles, and Kathrine felt so fresh she tacked another five miles for good measure.

Arnie, Kathrine, John Leonard from the cross-country team, and Kathrine's boyfriend, Tom Miller, entered the race, which had yet to adopt qualifying times. Kathrine signed her form K.V. Switzer, as usual, and got her number, 261, without any questioning.

"Boston was always Mecca for runners. Now I too was one of the anointed pilgrims," she wrote in her memoir, *Marathon Woman*.

The runners around her all seemed to think it was pretty neat that a girl was going to run. But not everyone was pleased to see her.

At mile four, a man grabbed Kathrine and tried to rip off her race number. It was Jock Semple, the president of the BAA, which organizes the race. A dust-up ensued, but Tom settled it. He left Jock crumpled by the side of the road. They all took off.

I can't imagine running a marathon with an adrenaline spike like that, but it got worse: Kathrine and Tom had an argument on the course, and Tom took off up ahead but later slowed to a walk. Kathrine passed him; she knew she had to keep going, or else everyone would believe she was just in it for the publicity.

So much goes through one's mind during a marathon, and for one of the first female marathoners, it was no different. Kathrine realized she wasn't special, running Boston, just lucky. All that women didn't have—teams and coaches and scholarships—wasn't necessarily because they didn't want it. They never even had the opportunity to demonstrate their desire.

John and Kathrine let Arnie finish just head of them. Nobody clapped for them, but reporters asked lots of questions. Someone told them their time was 4 hours, 20 minutes. Tom finished, too, eventually. They all drove back to Syracuse. K.V. Switzer was on the front page of all the newspapers the next day.

But still, nothing was different. Women were still banned from the race in 1968, and the year after that, and so on.

But now that women were going the distance, they weren't about to stop, even if the Boston Marathon refused to recognize their participation as legitimate. The BAA now calls the years 1966–1971 as the "pre-sanctioned" era of the Boston Marathon.

When researching all this, it's hard for me to wrap my head around women being excluded from the Boston Marathon or being forced to run it on the sly. At the same time, though, it's not that hard to imagine; people, most of them men, still laugh and yell crude things at me when I'm minding my own business, jogging around Portland decades later.

In 1972, a woman named Nina Kuscsik successfully petitioned The Amateur Athletics Union (AAU) to change the rules governing distances for women, which allowed the Boston Marathon to become a sanctioned race for women for the first time that year. It was the second year the Boston Marathon required runners to submit a qualifying time to gain entry to the race, and the qualifying time for women was the same as the men: 3 hours and 30 minutes.

Nina became the winner of the first official Boston Marathon women's race. Eight months later, I was born. It's incredible to think that women's distance racing is about the same age as me. But for a baby of a sport, it's got some incredible stories—ones that will inspire me on my runs.

CHAPTER ELEVEN

Nothing New in Little Beirut

IN THE 1990S, protestors greeted President George H. W. Bush whenever he came to Portland. They were so reliably rowdy that the president's staffers nicknamed the city Little Beirut. The name stuck, delighting activists, who took it as official recognition they'd become a thorn in the president's side. Mission accomplished.

The more things change, the more they stay the same. It's October 2004, and Mom and I have just checked into the Portland Hilton, where the first President Bush stayed on trips to Little Beirut. His son, George W., is running for his second term as president. If voters re-elect him and he returns to Portland, he'll no doubt be greeted by some of the people who protested him during his last term as president and his father before that.

But today, rather than filled with protestors, the Little Beirut Hilton is filled with runners. They're easy to identify, in shirts and jackets with names of marathons on them. Meanwhile, my blank shirt screams non-partisan. I feel like I've infiltrated a convention for a political party of which I'm not a member.

I'm staying at this particular hotel, as several months ago I moved from Portland to Seattle, making me feel like even more of an outsider. Moreover, marathon training now feels like it's a holdover from another life when I was driving around giving out books. When I lived in the apartment on Yamhill Street and every day was sweltering.

It's damp and chilly and gets dark early now, in Seattle, where I live.

Book giveaway is over. In late summer, I accepted a job at a newspaper in the Seattle suburbs.

I drove up to interview with Kevin, the editor, who was tan and as chubby-cheeked as a baby. He looked so sleepy that I thought he might nod off during our interview. He described in detail the company's Employee Assistance Plan, and how helpful it was when he was having trouble with his son. Of the newspaper's coverage, or what he'd like to see improved, he said almost nothing at all. No matter—it was a job in journalism, in the Seattle area, home to Dan and my mom. I wasn't going to pass it up.

The company refers to their publications as community newsweeklies. Essentially, the paper is a weekly but not an alternative weekly. In fact, there's no alternative: People in the community get the paper delivered to them whether they subscribe to it or not, making them a captive audience for advertisers. For this reason, some employees and readers in the community refer to it as a "shopper."

My new co-workers seem friendly, yet deferential. One of them tells me Kevin described me as a "veteran" reporter. I try to hide my amusement. Everything is relative. And though he looked to be barely staying awake, Kevin managed to fill an entry-level job with someone with years of experience, so really, the joke is on me.

In any case, I'm thrilled to be back in a regular job, creating a new daily routine. I drive to work instead of taking the bus, and each morning, when I turn the key in the ignition, it's as if the pistons inside me are once again firing. I have somewhere to go. Finally, I am going somewhere.

Crossing the I-90 bridge that spans the shimmering waters of Lake Washington, I marvel at how much the entire area has changed. In the years I have lived elsewhere, the Puget Sound region has experienced tremendous growth. Shiny new skyscrapers dot the Seattle skyline, and streets bustle with prosperous-looking people and fancy new cars.

I've never run in Seattle before. Marathon training gets me to see a familiar place in a new way. As the marathon approached, my runs started to get shorter, like hours of daylight. I was able to do some of them on my lunch break, which seemed to calm my new-job nerves. Running, once an obligation, has become familiar, a comfort. It's one of the few things in my life that hasn't changed. A lot else seems up in the air, though.

But at the moment, I'm back in Portland for the pre-race ritual known as packet pick-up. I take an odd-looking escalator to the basement ballroom. It appears to have been repurposed from a now-defunct department store. The Bush men and their entourages probably took the elevator. More secure and presidential.

Once in the pickup area, volunteers pull alphabetized manila envelopes from cardboard filing boxes. I accept my packet with both hands, as if handling something fragile. Then I am pointed in the direction of the line for the finisher's t-shirt. The finisher's shirt already? I feel foolish and disappointed. All this time, I assumed you get your finisher's shirt at the finish line. It's a bummer to discover this isn't the case.

After picking up race numbers, shirts, and a "goody bag," we are funneled into an adjoining ballroom. Like the gift shop you are forced to walk through to exit any tourist trap, race organizers have set us up with no way out but through the expo, a type of trade show aimed at race participants and, to a lesser extent, the friends, partners, and children of race participants.

The hall is filled with running items. There are energy drinks and nutritional supplements and all sorts of products related to running, or bragging about running, or recovering from injuries sustained while running.

Racks of t-shirts and hats bear an array of jokey sayings: "Will run for wine," "I don't chase boys—I pass them," and "Start slowly, and taper off from there."

There are also bumper stickers which contain nothing but those all-important numbers: 26.2 and 13.1. The "miles" part is left out; it's assumed for those in the know. If the numbers don't make sense, then the sticker isn't meant for you.

Clumps of people gather around some exhibitor tables. A summer spent giving books away has honed my instincts for crowd behavior. Whenever there is a mass of people, there are free samples to be had.

I move towards the crowd to see what's being given out. I wait my turn for a slice of a "nutrition bar" that looks like chocolate but tastes like a cross between chalk and plastic. To add to its grossness, it's as chewy as jerky. I want to spit it out but there's no garbage can, so I look around for some water to wash it down. Paper cups of pale pink liquid are lined up on a nearby table, like shots on a bar. I grab a cup and knock it back. It's effervescent, like Alka-Seltzer, with a faint fake flavor that reminds me of the plastic berries my grandmother used to keep in a bowl on her coffee table.

It isn't enough, so I grab another.

"It's good, isn't it?" says a smiling young woman in a pink polo shirt. Flashing a tight-lipped smile, in case I have shards of carob in my teeth, I nod.

"Mmm… Delicious."

***

FEARFUL OF NOT waking up in time to get to the start on the morning of the Marathon, I set two alarms before going to bed, but instead, I sleep fitfully, sweating in the hot, dry, hotel-room air. On the first trill of the hotel phone wake-up call, I pop out of bed, wide-awake, feverish, heart racing. My mom is in the other queen bed, sleeping like a baby. It's middle-of-the-night dark outside, but today is the day.

I shower and then slather myself in Body Glide, a lubricant designed to prevent chafing. I eat a bagel smeared with butter. It tastes good. I would like to have another. Even more, I would like to crawl back into bed with a bag of bagels and the remote control.

Maybe I no longer want to run a marathon, or maybe I never actually did. Maybe I only want to *have* done it. *Welp*, either way, it's time to put up or shut up.

The start line is right outside the hotel. Dan meets me in the lobby, and we wait until it's time to line up. I want to be quiet, to sit down for a bit and save my legs, which tire easily when standing. Working odd retail jobs in high school revealed the extent of this tendency. I would have rather spent hours walking the floor of the store than trapped behind a cash register, legs aching.

Dan's sister, Catherine, is also running the marathon, but it's not her first marathon; she's run several of them before. When I see her, she's talking with her seventy-something grandmother, both standing on the hard faux-marble floor like it's comfortable as a cloud. With a beatific smile, Grandma surveys the lobby as if it's the most wonderful, fascinating sight.

I find an out-of-the-way spot on the stairway up to the mezzanine and plop down on the ornately patterned carpet. There is nothing to do or say before the gun goes off. Dan understands. We sit in silence.

Finally, Catherine motions to us; it's time. Runners start to empty the lobby. Outside, the streets are packed with people, cordoned off with metal fencing. We wind our way around the barriers until finally there's clearing where we can gather in the street. I can no longer see Catherine. I'm alone in a sea of people. But she's going to run faster, she probably wants to start up ahead.

Crammed with runners among the tallest downtown buildings, the sounds echo, making Portland feel like a much larger, crowded city. Runners crush together inside the metal fences set up along the street.

Many around me are wearing their Portland Marathon 2004 shirt, which exclaims FINISHER in all caps. It seems unlikely that so many, having trained for months, would've forgotten to bring a shirt to wear. Maybe wearing the race shirt is a tradition, and it's the reason they hand them out early?

I tried on all sorts of clothing before I finally settled on my race-day outfit: a pale pink New Balance tank top with black trim and black New Balance shorts. It was a splurge; I paid full retail price at the New Balance store in a fancy mall. I dutifully tried it all out during a "dress rehearsal" long run, per the runner's rule: Nothing new on race day.

Portland Fit coaches repeated this like a mantra throughout my training, and it's ingrained in me. Anything you intend to eat, wear, or use in this race should be practiced in advance. If you buy anything at the expo, don't wear it. Even the Body Glide you smear on your skin should be tested beforehand. It could go wrong. You might find you are allergic to the ingredients, or that it doesn't really Glide, and instead slides off when you sweat. Everything has to be tested before race day. Runners are urged to minimize the number of unknowns and control circumstances as much as humanly possible. Of course, not all circumstances can be anticipated, but having your clothing chafe because you didn't bother to try it out isn't one of them.

I buy into this philosophy, even when the advice seems like overkill.

I've tried out everything; the clothes I'm wearing, the Body Glide I've smeared on my skin, the flavor of Gatorade in my bottles. Still, I've been turning the phrase over like a pebble in my pocket: Nothing new on race day. For first-time marathoners like myself, it is a paradox: *Everything* is new on race day. How can it be any other way?

Some more experienced runners put it another way: "Control the controllables." It's a less elegant turn of phrase, but at least it acknowledges that some things are out of our hands.

When I first joined Portland Fit, my life felt utterly lacking in "controllables." Where I worked, whether I stayed in Portland or moved to another city, all of it felt subject to the whims of others. Training for a marathon has given me a chance to be in complete control of at least one aspect of my life.

The sky is overcast and grey, as if the sun has not fully risen. I feel as if I'm not entirely up, either. *Maybe this is the way to start a marathon, half-asleep, so you don't overthink it.* It's like the old Irish saying: May you be in heaven an hour before the devil knows you're dead.

A few people are saying something over the loudspeaker. I'd figured there'd just be a starting gun or an air horn and we'd all take off running, but there's a preamble to this constitution. A woman begins singing the national anthem into the microphone. Several runners around me doff their caps and put their hands on their hearts, so I do the same. It's like the start of a baseball game, except instead of being fans in the stands, I'm on the field today, a player.

With the national anthem, a wavering woman's voice singing it, all the people around me fervently standing at attention, the excitement I'd anticipated is finally coming over me.

Soon I hear the *pop* of the starting gun—*Play Ball!*—but thanks to my half marathon experience, I'm not fooled; I stay put. Gradually, people in front of me begin shuffling, and I join in, pressing the button on my watch as I cross the start mat, in unison with hundreds of others, in a symphony of tiny beeps.

The breathing of runners, countless inhalations and exhalations, are all around me. Underneath all this is a steady rhythm of footfalls, keeping time like a bassline. It's a strange soundtrack, at once intimate and anonymous, and it reminds me that, even as we runners set out together, we are each so alone.

We move through the downtown streets quickly. Already, I feel I'm running a little too fast, but I can't seem to slow down; I'm surfing the wave of runners coming behind me.

We enter the red Chinatown Gate to the steady thunder of Taiko drums, complete a loop along the waterfront of the Willamette River, and zigzag through the trendy residential neighborhood of Northwest Portland. Clumps of bundled-up people crowd alongside the tree-lined streets, cheering.

Some carry homemade signs, magic marker on poster board, offering encouragement to family and friends. The spectators seem sincerely excited by what we are doing. None of the signs show even a hint of sarcasm. It's as if someone had created an irony-free zone of America's most ironic city.

Every couple miles a pop-up awning creates a temporary stage. Rock bands play upbeat oldies. *I'm walking on sunshine, whoa-ohhh* . . .

Big wheel keep on turnin', proud Mary keep on burnin'. . .

It's a nice day for a white wedding, it's a nice day to . . .

A salsa band jams, and runners swivel their hips. People around me seem to perk up and surge a bit when they hear the bands, rushing by the music rather than slowing to savor it. I can't help but think how odd it must be to play to an audience that is constantly passing you by.

We stream past Montgomery Park, the former home of Montgomery Ward, a department store and mail order catalog company. The building was repurposed into a sprawling office complex in the 1980s. I did a stint as a temp at a big corporation with offices in the building, which looked as if they hadn't been updated since the 1890s. The work was monotonous, an unending string of data entry into Excel spreadsheets. On sunny days, the wide windows that look out over the city seemed to taunt me with all that I was missing. Even though there is no sunshine now, to be on the other side of those windows feels like an achievement. Once it became clear I could make far more money just giving away books, I left that gig, and now I have a permanent job as a reporter at a newspaper.

So long, temp work. Farewell Montgomery Park!

Leaving this location in the dust, I feel . . . good. Yeah, I can say that. I am putting Montgomery Park behind me.

A little farther up, a friend from my Portland Fit group, Ann, will be waiting. She's going to jump in and run with me. Ann, a native of Maine, always wears a Boston Red Sox cap when she runs, her curly brown hair exploding out the back. She is a veteran of several marathons, including this one, and has a sassy confidence that I admire. Ann is a few years older than me, married. She and her husband, Eric, and their adopted greyhound, Lucy, live in an old house in Southeast Portland that Eric is restoring. Ann has her act together. She is working on her PhD in mathematics at Portland State University and doesn't seem like the type to take crap from anybody. All this time I've spent running with her, I have hoped Ann's confidence and competence might rub off on me.

She spots me, hops in, and we run side-by-side down the highway. It's just like our long runs, rambling along the Willamette River.

By now the crowds of runners have strung out. The sky is overcast and dim. We don't talk much, this is serious business, but to have Ann beside me makes each step seem easier. She knows about pacing marathons. She knows this course. I don't have to think, just follow her and run.

I train my eyes into the middle distance, at the muscled calves of runners ahead of me. The view around me seems to be changing ever so slowly, or maybe not at all. My mind might be rewinding the miles and playing them over again.

Long gone are the kids with their high fives and hand-lettered signs. We've moved into an industrial area; no one would cheer on the sidelines here. The shoulder of the highway is muddy and dotted with litter. Is this really the course for a marathon?

I tried to break down the Portland Marathon course and run each part of it, piece by piece. I'd planned to run over the bridge and to the part we're covering now, so I drove from my apartment in Southeast Portland to the east side of the bridge. But I wasn't able to continue because the bridge sidewalks were closed during a thirty-eight-million-dollar rehabilitation project that wouldn't be completed for another year.

Now I see the part I didn't cover is the least attractive, most industrial segment of the course. The St. Johns Bridge must be up ahead, but it seems to be taking an awfully long time for it to come into view.

"Where is it, Ann?" I say, exasperated. "Where is the bridge?"

"It's right there, Amy," Ann replies, pointing straight ahead.

Emerging from the fog like a gothic dragon, the St. Johns Suspension

Bridge spans 2,000 feet across Willamette River. Built in 1929, its steel spires are Statue of Liberty green and impossible to miss unless, like me, you have your head down, staring at the pavement.

At the bridge's mid-span we will hit mile 19, but getting all the way up there will surely demand even more from my legs. And Ann won't be able to come with me.

Up ahead runners are making a sharp right onto the bridge. A race official or volunteer is stationed at the approach, checking runners for bib numbers. A sign says only runners with race numbers will be allowed to continue.

The road is steeper now. We're ascending to the approach of the bridge. People around me start to slow, and some began to walk. Ann keeps striding confidently, so I do the same.

"This is where I say goodbye," she says.

I want to grab Ann and beg her not to go. It feels like we've been on a training run and everything has been fine. When she's gone, it'll be a marathon, the real thing, and I'll be on my own. Ann would probably run the whole marathon with me, just for practice. But the course marshal up ahead is seeing to it that no one who isn't registered gets onto the bridge.

So this is it. Ann is steps behind already.

"Thanks, Ann!" I holler and wave. I hope I sound grateful, not fearful.

I'm not sure she can hear me, anyway. A lone drummer is stationed near the point where we step on the bridge, slapping the skins solemnly. The beat is a reminder to keep moving my feet, in short, quick steps, trying to keep up my cadence. The bridge is steep, I try not to look too far ahead. It seems we're climbing to the sky.

The arch of my left foot is numb now. Apparently, it's fallen asleep. It's weird and unnerving, but my foot is still doing its job. I'm continuing to slam it against concrete, so it will probably "wake up" eventually.

As I hit the midpoint of the bridge, I look west over the city. The bridge sways in the wind. All of Portland is laid out before me, buildings set on curt little blocks, cars small as ants, scurrying around downtown. Far below, brown water is flowing, the Willamette River as I've never seen her.

Rio Vista, I think, smiling to myself.

Few people get to see Portland from this vantage point, and best of all, I've earned it. This morning, for a few hours, Portland's bridges and streets belong to people on foot, not in cars. Some runners stop to take pictures, as if merely sightseeing, not marathoning. I didn't bring a camera, so I keep going, relieved as the course tips downhill, my legs picking up speed.

It's too steep to run comfortably. My quads shudder as I press down on the brakes. Toward the end of the bridge, a photographer is crouched, clicking a shutter full of runners. When I get to him, I try to pull myself together and smile.

The hardest part of the course is behind us, or so I've been told. After the bridge, the course undulates along a bluff, near the campus of the University of Portland. This part should be a lucky area, since my mother, aunt, and brother, Matt, are alumni of the school, Matt having run for the school's track and cross-country teams. As he predicted, several of the school's athletes, some of whom live in shared housing along the course, are out in their university gear, looking fresh-faced and enthusiastic. It gives me a lift to see the Pilots in their purple.

But as soon as they're out of my sight, a fog comes over me. I'm trudging along a bluff on a lovely tree-lined street, unable to appreciate the scenery. The *wow-I'm-running-a-marathon* feeling has disappeared, replaced by a dull ache in my legs. I'm hoping that I didn't hit a wall.

Just past mile 19, Daniel is waiting. He spots me first and jogs next to me in his plaid shirt and jeans, offering encouragement. Seeing him running comfortably in regular clothing while I am all kitted out in running gear, demonstrates just how slow I'm going. At least Ann can't see me now.

"I can't talk," I say, preemptively. I want to absorb Daniel's energy without expending any of my own.

But less than a quarter-mile away is a sight to behold: members of my Portland Fit group have assembled a pep rally on the course, complete with a massive arch of yellow and red balloons and speakers blaring disco music. They wear yellow-and-red t-shirts, the group's signature colors, and some wave pom-poms. They line up along the route, each holding out a hand for a high five.

Transformed by the sight, I surge toward the line of people, whooping as I slap hands, one after another, down the entire line.

Where did this energy come from? It's as if someone had flipped a switch. Was this the girl who, just moments earlier, had told her boyfriend she was too tired to speak? If I do I have something left, it's time to use it up.

And I do—all of it. I'm not elated, or proud, or joyful in the least as I cross the finish line of the 2004 Portland Marathon, 4 hours, 23 minutes, and 23 seconds after I started.

I feel . . . nothing. I shuffle past volunteers who hand things to me, a bottle of water, a bag of food, a finisher's medal around my neck. I don't want any of it. I want to lie down, to cease to exist. I would like to sip from a tall, cool glass of nothingness.

A volunteer hands me a bag and tells me there is a tree inside of it. I just ran the Arbor Day Marathon, apparently. I take the tree, a seedling, technically, and keep moving, as everyone is encouraging us to do. More runners are coming in behind us; race officials don't want a bottleneck.

Once I get through the fenced-off area, Dan and Mom find me. I try to smile, but I'm at a loss for words. Someone finally takes the tree from me, as well as all the random items I've been struggling to carry.

The Hilton is one of the hotels closest to the finish, but right now, it is so far. I can barely lift my legs along the sidewalk. Every move is feeble, like I'm one hundred years old. Getting down off the curb and back up requires help from Daniel. Mom has a worried look. She's talking, asking questions. I hardly answer, though I know I should. My silence is probably more worrying to her than any complaint I could make.

In the hotel, I shower and change. I put on my too-big finisher's shirt because, finally, it's not false advertising. I am a marathon finisher. I put the medal back on, too. It's enormous, fit for a champion, or Mr. T.

Mom and I slowly make our way to Mother's, a restaurant I'd picked out beforehand, where Daniel is waiting. My feet are swollen and tender, my joints stiff, but I no longer feel like a centenarian. More like age ninety-five. On the sidewalk, people smile and congratulate me, and I do the same in return. In our identical blue shirts and dangling golden medallions, I feel ridiculous, yet happily oblivious, like an adult trick-or-treater on Halloween.

My friend Kristy, who was there for my first half marathon four months ago, has already gotten us a table for us at Mother's. I order their famous crunchy French toast and coffee, delicious coffee. The food comes quickly and is the perfect combination of salty, sweet, crunchy, and soft, the richness of the coffee burnished by cream. Caffeinated and, finally, knee-deep in present hedonism, I could go on all day about the flavors I'm experiencing.

The restaurant staff and people at nearby tables smile at me and offer their congratulations. I thank them and smile and congratulate back. Yay for all of us, marathon finishers! Mimosas all around. Mother's is a Portland institution, but this is the best breakfast I've ever had anywhere, not just for the food, but also because it seems the whole restaurant is celebrating a holiday with me. *Viva la marathon!*

On the way back to Seattle, I lay down in the back seat and fall asleep somewhere on I-5. Dan is driving with Mom beside him in the passenger seat. When I wake up, all I can see is the back of their heads framed by the sunset; the morning cloud cover burned off to a blue-sky day fading to indigo. We stop at Burgerville for milk shakes. They are thick and rich, and as I spoon mine out, I am no longer ancient-feeling. I'm a ten-year-old who just got her tonsils out.

I never saw Catherine after the race; she finished far ahead of me, in 3:39:02.

It wasn't until a few days later that I learned it was her fastest marathon, a personal record (PR), and a Boston qualifying time (BQ). The Boston Marathon of my memory—colorfully dressed runners cramming onto the subway; grandstands set up in front of the Boston Public Library—is just up ahead of her now.

Some people in the green group had been talking about running the marathon in four hours, a solid time for a time-timer. I must've started out running with some of them, although that was not my intention. At the 10K mark, I was averaging 9:28 minutes per mile, but I slowed down. By the halfway point, I was at 9:36 per mile, and then, after I saw Daniel, I slowed even more, to an average pace of 9:52.

Like the bumper sticker says, start slowly, and taper off from there. All told, I averaged 9:58 per mile, a long way from the four-hour marathon pace of 9:01 per mile. Not that it matters. I finished.

It feels like a lifetime ago that I started training for the Portland

Marathon. And it feels like a lifetime I lived inside of the 26.2 miles I ran today. But I've caught the marathon bug, and I'm not about to stop here.

To qualify for the Boston Marathon, as Catherine has done, I must improve my performance by 43 minutes and 23 seconds. Put another way, I must speed up from a 9:58-per-mile pace to an 8:19 pace.

I looked up my Boston Marathon qualifying time one summer day, fatigued from a long run that morning and seeking inspiration. It's the era of dial-up internet, so the list of qualifying times and age groups takes forever to appear. I nearly laughed out loud when it finally did load. Three hours and forty minutes seemed far-fetched, ridiculous.

Now I've run a marathon, but this attitude hasn't changed. The Boston Marathon is still a lifetime away.

CHAPTER TWELVE

Joanie

It's Friday after the marathon. I've been sore and happy for the last four days. Now it's time for a celebration, but not for me.

Mr. Silicon Valley is flying me and many others to San Francisco to attend a Saturday-night party he's throwing in honor of our success at handing out his novel. Apparently, we've done a laudable job pressing hundreds of thousands of copies into the hands of the unsuspecting. His company is taking care of all the travel arrangements. I was told to keep the receipts for any expenses; I'll be reimbursed for them.

I feel a bit disingenuous taking the trip, given my feelings about the book. And I suspect many of the books I gave away never got read and ended up in a dumpster. Well, hopefully they ended up in a Goodwill donation bin, or at least, recycling. *Wait, can you recycle a hardcover book?*

It's not like it would've changed anything if I hadn't taken his money. The books were already printed; they had to go somewhere. I did exactly what I was paid to do—put them in the hands of people who might read them. It's not my fault if no one follows through.

Besides, the trip is a chance to see my college friend Maryrose, who is coming up from LA to be my date for the party. I've told her about the book job, and she agrees it's weird but has never been one to look a gift horse in the mouth. Our plan is to make an appearance and smile, grateful the largesse of the Silicon Valley economy trickles down to liberal arts majors like us.

Maryrose's flight isn't due in until late morning, but I get up early Saturday. My marathon experience still fresh in my mind, I brought my running clothes with me. I'm somewhat familiar with San Francisco, having taken the train into the city from Stanford on several occasions during grad school, and I was eager to see it in a new way.

It's the first time I've run since the Portland Marathon. For two days, it was difficult to walk, but that's over now. I'm walking normally, so I hope I'll be running normally, too.

I step into the classic San Francisco weather, with a marine layer of clouds that will burn off later.

"The fog comes in on little cat feet."

I always think of this line from the Carl Sandburg poem when I see San Francisco, which I now realize has the perfect running weather: cool in the mornings, yet mild enough for short sleeves and shorts.

My plan is to run down to the Embarcadero and just turn around whenever I get tired. Coincidentally, as I head across Union Square, I see people setting up for what looks like, yes, a marathon. It's the Nike Women's Marathon. Runners are standing outside the Nike store.

I had no idea it was happening this weekend. A few of them notice me in my running gear. They are going on a pre-race run; do I want to join?

Emboldened by my newly-minted marathoner status, I say yes.

But oh, man, what have I agreed to?

A television crew has set up on the sidewalk filming the crowd. I try to stay out of the camera. This is pre-race coverage, but I'm not among the race participants. In fact, I'm not even sure how far I can run today. I might still be recovering from my own marathon.

We pick up more people; safety in numbers. I was worried that I wouldn't be able to keep up, but there are at least twenty of us now, and on city streets, it will be impossible for us to run quickly.

We take off toward the waterfront, running way more slowly than I expected, almost gently. We are creeping around the city on little cat feet.

From the conversation around me, I glean that this is what's known as a "shakeout," something I didn't do a week ago, before Portland, because I'd never even heard of such a thing. Everyone is saving their legs for tomorrow's race.

Runners are chatting excitedly amongst themselves, all of them women.

Are any men entered in the Nike Women's Marathon?

Next to me is a statuesque twentysomething who happens to be from Mercer Island, an affluent suburb of Seattle. She tells me it's the inaugural edition of the race and some celebrities are here for it, including Joan Benoit Samuelson. The woman says the name like it's nothing.

Wait, what? Joan Benoit Samuelson, the winner of the first Olympic women's marathon, in 1984? Two-time winner of the Boston Marathon?

I'm dumbstruck as I search my own mind for how I know about Joan Benoit Samuelson. Is it because I've always watched the Olympics?

Another runner overhears us talking and whispers to me, "She's right there!"

Joanie, as she is known, is running a few feet in front of me. If I reach out my arm, I could touch her back. She is a small woman with short salt-and-pepper hair under a white Nike cap. She's practically swimming in her boxy white t-shirt and baggy black running shorts. Her presentation is so nondescript, it's almost like she doesn't want to be recognized.

It is hard for me to believe this is the same woman I've seen in historical footage, winning at the Olympics.

I don't begrudge the runners around me for not knowing all the past winners of the Boston Marathon, but women marathoners who don't know the winner of the first Olympic women's marathon?

I'm not angry; just disappointed.

When Joanie first won Boston, with a time of 2:35:15, it was a new American record and seven minutes faster than any woman had ever run Boston before. Winning in Los Angeles, in 1984, is what made Joanie a household name. It was the first time there'd ever been a women's marathon at the Olympic Games. She'd had knee surgery just two weeks earlier. When she made her move, at mile 22, no one went with her. Joanie ran alone the rest of the way, with no one in sight as she entered the tunnel of the Olympic stadium and onto the track to win the first gold medal in the women's event.

Now the legend is right in front of me; smaller than life. She's so soft-spoken that I can't even hear what she is saying, but she seems to be listening more than talking. That makes sense; Joanie is from Maine, and from what I know of northern New Englanders, they follow the Ben Franklin rule of avoiding trifling conversation.

But because I'm from the West Coast, and trained as a journalist, I can't help but think people ought to be taking advantage of the opportunity to ask her questions, learn from her. Isn't that why she's here?

I search for something to ask Joanie. Had I known I'd be running with her I would've prepared some questions. Her back is to me, so it'd be hard to ask them, anyway.

Joanie must be in her fifties now and is still competing as a master, the category for athletes age forty and over. Maybe this slight, unassuming, no-nonsense woman is over talking about herself, or her career, or was never into it to begin with. Perhaps she is simply happy to run amid a bunch of babbling recreational runners who are excited to run a marathon tomorrow, maybe their first.

I look down at her feet. Her legs are very thin and pale, and she's wearing Nike running shoes and white socks that are just a tad too long to be fashionable.

The women around her are in full faces of makeup, as if they anticipated part of this run might be televised, and bright, head-to-toe Nike clothing. I wonder if Joanie enjoys running with a bunch of strangers, all wanting to be in proximity but not having anything meaningful to say.

The gap between us is a wide chasm; me a recreational amateur and a brand-new one at that, and she a running legend, a professional who has dedicated her life to the sport. Yet, by chance, on the streets of San Francisco, we are running together. Well, if not actually "together," then in close proximity.

What could Joan Benoit Samuelson and I have in common? Nothing, of course. And then again, we have running in common. It's something.

As we finish, I wish the runners near me good luck on their races, and jog back across Union Square, now dotted with tents set up as part at the race staging. In front of them are tall bar tables covered with linens. Squares of Ghirardelli chocolate, a race sponsor, have been arranged on the tables, reminding me of medals.

I wonder where Joan keeps her gold medal from the Olympics. I can't imagine her pretending to bite into it for a photo, like people do today.

I grab a couple of the shiny, foil-wrapped squares, one for myself, and one for Maryrose. I didn't earn these, but I'm taking them anyway.

When I burst into the room, Maryrose has just arrived and is getting settled in.

"Don't you look sporty," she says, in her half-teasing, half-sincere way.

"Welcome to San Francisco," I say, tossing her a square of chocolate.

We hug hello, and I tell her all about my new running buddy, an Olympic Gold Medalist, as we eat our chocolate for breakfast.

CHAPTER THIRTEEN
The Wall of Death

A MONTH AFTER the Portland Marathon, I ran the Seattle Half Marathon. Along the course, I noticed runners crowding around a runner holding numbered signs. They were pace group leaders, and each of them wore a vest emblazoned with the word "Chuckit."

I can figure out what a pace group is—that is self-explanatory. But what the heck is Chuckit? I Google it to find it's a brand of dog toy, as well as a local running club coached by a man named Chuck Bartlett. Sounds more like a club for people who like to throw things, but whatever.

Nevertheless, the name sticks in my head, which was probably the point behind the odd name. One cold Wednesday evening in January, I kill an hour after work, waiting until time to show up at a running store for one of Chuckit's weekly workouts.

The atmosphere in the store is nowhere near as relaxed and casual as Portland Fit. Serious-looking runners clad in tights, technical shirts and vests and with large, important-looking watches strapped to their wrists stretch their quads confidently on the hardwood floor of the store. The store is in a new, mixed-use development. Bright track lights illuminate all the latest running gear for sale. I could leave, but more people are coming in, blocking the door. In this small space, it's going to be impossible to exit unnoticed.

A fit-looking woman in black running gear is discussing her workout with the man I determined to be Chuck, her pale ponytail bobbing as she nods in understanding. I can't quite make out their conversation, but it appears serious, as if he's a surgeon and she's his patient.

Chuck's coaching career was built on a formidable running resume that started with track and cross-country championships in high school and continued in college and beyond. He was an All-American in Cross Country at Adams State College, a storied distance program built by the legendary coach Joe Vigil. When Chuck took to the roads after graduating, he triumphed there, too, running a marathon PR of 2:19 in the Seattle Marathon.

When the woman Chuck is talking to leaves, I introduce myself and say I've just run the Portland Marathon.

"What was your time?"

I tell him: 4:23:23. Chuck says nothing, shows no expression. Maybe I should've told him my new half marathon time (1:54:30) instead? Someone calls his name, and without another word, Chuck turns and walks away.

Huh. I'd expected simply having completed a marathon would have earned me a little credibility. Now that seems naïve.

My stomach is queasy.

Maybe coming here is a mistake.

Before I can even think of leaving, Chuck starts to talk. Runners form a semi-circle around him. He describes how to do tonight's workout: bound up the hills, slowly, but with knees thrust high in the air. The second time, it's slightly faster, and with a less exaggerated form. Finally, we'll run normally, hard up the hill. These three repeats constitute one "set."

People exit the store and set out along the sidewalk. It's now or never. I fall in behind the last person. A few blocks away, we arrive at the designated place to do our hill repeats. It's a long, four-lane road that leads straight up a gradual hill, part of a busy street lined with apartments and condos.

The neighborhood is unfamiliar to me, as is this workout. In Portland Fit, whenever we encountered hills on our runs, we simply went up them—once.

I mimic the other runners, trailing them and trying not to fall too far behind. The high knees thing feels goofy.

I'm not sure what exaggerating the motion of running is supposed to accomplish. But I'm a 4:23 marathoner, what do I know?

We "recover" on the jog back down and regroup at the bottom of the hill, where Chuck has stationed himself, arms folded across his chest, casting an appraising eye on each of us as we appear and retreat.

Even though I do it slowly, the jog back down the hill doesn't leave me feeling fully rested for the run back up. Fatigue is starting to pile up. By the time we've completed the set, about thirty minutes have passed. I'm exhausted. And we have one more set to go. On the way back to the store, Chuck runs past me. "Not bad, buddy," he says, "You're stronger than I thought."

It's a backhanded compliment, but still, it's a relief. I'm not the fastest runner on those hills, not by a long shot. Just the same, I am in the club.

On Saturdays, Chuckit meets for long runs at the uncivilized hour of 7:30 a.m. I doubt there'll be much of a turnout when I set out to meet them on this cold, dark winter morning. When I get to the meeting place, a Seattle running store, the lights are off. I turn the knob anyway, and the door swings open. It's unlocked.

Reflective accents on running clothing glint like the beady eyes of animals in a forest. It's not even dawn, but dozens of people are here, standing around in the dark.

Chuck approaches and introduces me to some of the other members. I'm definitely the new kid on the block. I squint as my eyes adjust to the low light.

A half-dozen people are going on an eight-mile run, a distance that sounds manageable. After a brief homily from Chuck, I set out with them into the cold, cloudy morning.

I find myself running behind a young woman in black running tights with stylish gold piping down the legs and a matching black jacket. Her glossy dark hair is pulled into a ponytail, and a black headband covers her ears. Although I recognize the signature swoosh, her outfit is one you'd be hard-pressed to find at an outlet store. I didn't even know Nike made anything so stylish. Must be Nike Couture.

The wearer of such finery is Rachele, who appears to be leading this run. She tells everyone that should the group get strung out, we'll regroup at the Wall of Death.

Wait, did she just say wall of death? I envision an epic hill, steeper than the one we'd done our hill repeats on Wednesday night. And yet Rachele tosses it off casually; yes, we're running to the Wall of Death, no biggie.

Marathoners are always talking about "hitting the wall," but I've never heard anyone talk about a Wall of *Death.* Seems a little dramatic. Perhaps Wall of Death is an ironic joke, and it is barely even an incline. I very much hope that this is the case as we're running at a pace that's comfortable for me now, but one I likely wouldn't be able to maintain if forced to scale a Wall. Of. Death.

On the other hand, maybe the Wall of Death is something else entirely, like, the name of an edgy record store near the University of Washington: "Dude, the vinyl selection at Wall of Death is totally sick!"

There is no sense worrying and wondering about something that I have no control over. I'm going to push this wall from my mind. If I can just stay near Rachele, I won't need to recognize the wall at all.

The sun is up so the sky is a brighter shade of grey. We continue down the Burke-Gilman Trail, a paved bike path, which is empty of cyclists and dead flat. No walls, not a grim reaper in sight. We approach a bridge that spans Portage Bay, which connects Lake Union and Lake Washington. The water reflects the sky, blue-grey. A seagull lets out a plaintive cry.

Once underneath the bridge, Rachele and the others stop. It's warmer here, and we are out of the wind.

Grey-painted pikes stick up from the ground underneath the bridge, supporting a coral-colored ring sitting atop it like a crown. This appears to be a quirky work of public art. Out of sight under a bridge is sure an odd place to put it.

While we're waiting I just bend down and pretend to stretch my legs.

As I stand back up, I see it: Stenciled in black, blocky letters on the coral crown of the public art installation: "The Wall of Death."

This is The Wall of Death?

I nearly laugh out loud.

CHAPTER FOURTEEN

Ropes and Ladders

IT'S A DARK day at Sunny Hills Elementary. I'm in the second grade and feeling nervous. Today, my class is supposed to climb a rope up to the gymnasium's ceiling. Or at least, we are supposed to try. A thick, blue gymnastics pad has been placed on the ground underneath, in case someone falls.

A boy inches his body up the rope. My stomach is in knots. I can't be the only one who thinks that it's crazy we are being asked to do this. I'm a second-grader, not Spider-Man. But I don't have a choice.

When my turn comes, the rough, yellow coil scratches my tender fingers. *Owww*. Gripping it, knees bent, swaying from the bottom, I'm amazed anyone has the strength to pull themselves up.

I certainly don't; all I have is a tummy ache.

In the school nurse's office, I lay down on a cot covered in crinkly tissue paper and pray they don't call Mom. As soon as PE is over, I feel better. Like magic. Or like my prayers have been answered. A little of each, probably. Still, it's an experience that I won't soon forget.

In junior high, we have the privilege of choosing which PE class to take—the one with badminton, or the one with flag football. This ends up, predictably, with girls in the badminton class and boys in the other.

Three weeks later, the teacher tells us it's illegal.

Huh? Badminton is illegal?

No, the fact that all the girls are in one class, and the boys are in the other. Gender segregation, it's called.

Eventually, me and another girl, Pat, are moved to a class taught by the football coach that is otherwise full of boys, while two of the boys from that class are moved to the class we'd picked, which features non-contact sports like floor hockey and is taught by a woman. A little switcheroo and *voila!* Equality.

Our new teacher, Mr. E., is a well-known hard-ass who coaches football and wrestling and seems not the least bit pleased to have girls in his class. Welcome to the club; Pat and I don't want to be here, either. But what are we supposed to do? We're not adults. We didn't make the law.

A tall, strapping girl, Pat is an ace pitcher for the girls' softball team but quiet as a mouse. She tolerates PE's indignities with preternatural calm, while my seething contempt for Mr. E., and for this whole messed-up situation, is written all over my face. It's a tense few months.

In the spring, seventh graders take the Presidential Fitness test. Mostly, it doesn't sound too bad; it's made up of tasks like doing a certain number of sit-ups in a certain number of minutes, with Pat patiently holding down my feet, and the shuttle run, a pointless task of moving chalkboard erasers from one part of the gym to another.

But the final test is as frightening as rope-climbing from second grade. We have to run a mile, four long laps on the track. Our performance on this, and all the other tasks, is measured in percentiles, which, though I'm not great at math, I understand is the same as being graded on a curve. So, unlike most tests we take, where it's possible for everyone to earn an A, the whole point of the Presidential Fitness test is that not everyone will be able to pass.

Even at the young age of 12, I'm skeptical of Presidential Fitness. I know for a fact the current president, Ronald Reagan, eats jelly beans and falls asleep at his desk, so I highly doubt his physical fitness is the standard to which America's pre-teens ought to aspire.

Also, it's strange that the president of the country has a say in PE, but there's no presidential test for, say, math or social studies. I'm not prepared to go all-in on a test without a little context. *Please.*

But it's middle school. We haven't gotten to context yet. Mr. E. holds a stopwatch and yells (encouragement?) while the boys plus Pat and I set out for our four laps. The boys sprint up ahead. Pat and I run together. By the final lap, I'm so tired of Mr. E's hollering I speed up, leaving Pat behind.

Pat comes in last; all the boys are done. I feel bad, having dropped her, but as usual, Pat doesn't seem to mind. Why should she? Pat has no need for a patch with a bald eagle on it. She's a bona fide student-athlete, and if that doesn't count as presidentially-fit, then in my book, it's meaningless.

I'm practically done with PE anyway. When I join the swim team up at the high school, I'll be able to waive the physical education requirement. After that, I'll never have to set foot on a track again, if I don't want to.

And why on earth would I want to?

This is the same question now before me, some twenty years after the fact. The prospect of running on a track, especially with others around, is like taking a time machine back to junior high, or to the second-grade nausea I felt under the rope that I never climbed. (If I'm being honest, I never even tried to climb.)

But today is Tuesday, and on Tuesdays, Chuckit hits the track.

This is a new type of training for me. There were no track workouts in Portland Fit. Or maybe, more experienced runners did track workouts but were sworn to a kind of *Fight Club* silence: The first rule about track workouts is you don't talk about track workouts. Had I realized running on a track was part of training for a marathon, I probably would not have signed up for it. After all, the best thing about being an adult is that no one can make you do something you don't want to do.

The marathon, to me, represents a journey into the unknown, a solitary pursuit, man against nature, man against himself, not the stuff of seventh grade. But maybe what they say is true: Adult life is just high school, but with even more stuff you don't want to do.

We start out easy, jogging. The track is a mile from the running store where we meet, so we'll warm up on the way over. I don't recognize anybody from the hill workout, or the Saturday run to the Wall of Death.

I fall in behind the pack as we take over the gravel path around Green Lake. Runners make way for us, some of them turning their heads as we pass. I've picked the perfect day for my first track workout, someone says. It's the one day a month where Chuck has the two-mile time trial.

Great.

I'm not supposed to freak out about this. The point of the time trial is to establish a set point for your fitness, on which to peg your track workouts. It is not a test, but it sure feels like it.

The dirt track runs around a grass soccer field, with more soccer fields nearby. It is rutted and rocky. Someone has dragged a line in it to mark the start. Chuck holds a digital stopwatch to time us. We are going off in two groups, so I self-select into the second, slower group.

My heart is beating in my mouth now. Swallow, take a deep breath, and . . . *Go!*

A scuffling sound of feet slapping the dirt, kicking up dust. A few people sprint to get out in front and lead. Everyone cuts over toward the inside of the track, known as Lane One. There's no time to think, so I cut over to the inside, too, and try to close the gap between myself and the person just up ahead of me. I don't want to run a greater distance than I need to.

By the time we hit the first turn, we have sorted ourselves into a line. A few people run up on me from behind and fit their way in ahead of me. They're welcome to it; I'm working hard already and don't think that I can keep up.

Coming out of the turn, I remind myself to relax.

Two miles is how far? Eight laps. I want to be able to make it through all of them.

I feel awkward, uncertain how far I should kick out my legs, or how high should I pull up my knees. And how do I time this all with the breathing? Isn't running supposed to come naturally?

In the periphery of my vision, I can see Chuck on the other side of the soccer field. The lead runners are reaching him now. They are half a lap ahead already.

In front of me is a woman in teal-blue shorts. I concentrate on the color, teal-blue, like the ocean, a calm sea, clear sailing ahead. My breaths are short, sharp. I slow them down, exhaling completely as I focus on the blue of her shorts.

Nearing the line where we started, Chuck is calling out numbers as people pass him; reading times off his stopwatch.

"Good job, Buddy," he says as I reach him.

I guess that's me: Buddy. I guess I'm doing okay?

First lap down, seven to go.

Teal shorts is still right in front of me. Her steps are quick. She runs on her tippy-toes, as if there's barely time to set her whole foot on the ground before picking it up again. Her body is small and compact, straight to the point. Next to her, I feel oversized and awkward, a gangly, spasmodic try-hard, desperate to hang on, but I am hanging on.

For the third lap, and the fourth and fifth, I manage to stay close to teal shorts, careful not to step on her heels. That would be impossible anyway since she never seems to set them down.

How many laps left? I've lost count. A burning sensation spreads through the back of my thighs.

Teal shorts is pulling ahead. No, it's me; I'm falling behind.

Several people have lapped us now. They're finishing already. I'm overcome with a sickening uncertainty: *I might not make it.*

I'm not sure what is happening, but my legs are shaking. The track is emptying of runners. My arms, swinging at my sides, are the only limbs working properly. How to run no longer concerns me, I only hope to keep going.

There's fewer of us on the track, our breathing now seems amplified.

Here we are, on display. No. Banish the thought. Concentrate on teal shorts, right in my line of sight. Blue is a calming color, they use it on the walls of prisons and waiting rooms. Use the blue.

"Last lap," someone says, to my intense relief. I can see Chuck with his stopwatch, across the grassy field from me.

How many steps away is he? How many breaths left to breathe?

Suddenly and yet following eternity, I round the final bend, under the branches hanging low over the track, careful not to trip in the gaping pothole, and to the line in the sand. Chuck is next to it, with his stopwatch, but I am staring into the distance, framed by the brim of my cap. I pull my arms tight to my sides and fling my legs out ahead, long strides now, why I do not know. Just feels like the right thing to do.

"15:04," Chuck says as I cross the line.

Exhaustion. Relief.

I thought it was just me and teal shorts left running, but several people are coming in behind us. I'm not last, not even close. It feels so good to be finished. It's not like I'm skilled at running on the track. It's scary and difficult. But anyway, I did it.

Maybe the benefit of being an adult isn't refusing to do things because they tie your stomach in knots, but choosing to do them anyway, finding a way through, and enjoying the satisfaction that comes from having faced down your fears.

I don't have to like running on a track. I don't have to be good at it, even. All I need to do is all I've ever really needed to do: just *try*.

Now that I've run a time trial, I have a sense of the pace that I'm supposed to hit as I run, and, importantly, who I'm able to run those paces with. Novel as it is, each track workout feels like a big deal, bigger even than Saturday long runs. Monday nights, I pack a bag with my running clothes and shoes. I go to Chuckit straight after work, so I change before I get in the car.

The newspaper offices are in Bellevue, across Lake Washington from Green Lake, where Chuckit meets. This requires me to drive through one of the region's worst rush-hour traffic bottlenecks: over the Evergreen Point Floating Bridge, and then up Interstate 5. Every week, I gaze at the sea of red brake lights in front of me and wonder if I am going to make it.

Sometimes, I am so late I have to drive straight to the parking lot near the track, instead of parking near the store, missing the mile warm-up on the way over and jumping right into the workout in progress (not recommended).

Also, there is the problem of food. By the time we are to meet, at 6:30 p.m., I am starting to get hungry from lunch. I try to remember to bring an energy bar or something to eat on the drive, but one day, I forget.

My stomach rumbles as I sit in my car on the bridge, willing the traffic to roll forward.

This isn't good. By the time I find a parking spot near the running store, it's already time to meet. I'm annoyingly hungry, but there's no food store nearby, and I'm not about to move my car from my precious parking spot. But there is a Starbucks next to the running store. I walk in—no line, my lucky day—and order a chocolate chip cookie. Yes, just the cookie, no coffee. I'm in running gear, but the barista doesn't blink. I wait near the drinks station for him to give it to me. A man looks up from his phone: It's Chuck, waiting for his usual vanilla latte.

The barista hands me a white paper bag with the cookie inside.

"What ya got there?" Chuck says, smirking mischievously.

"It's a cookie," I say, feeling my face reddening. I could try to explain that I forgot my snack, that I usually don't eat cookies before a workout, that I had no time to stop at a store on the drive over, traffic, blah, blah, blah...

It's no use. Any explanation I might provide will be canceled out by what he sees: me ordering a cookie at Starbucks just minutes before a track workout.

Chuck is still waiting for his vanilla latte as I begin to leave.

"See you in a few," I say, slinking out of the store to eat my cookie in peace. Well, half the cookie. I'm going to save the other half for later. That was the plan, anyway. But I looked in the bag and found it empty. Without even knowing it, I had the last bite. I take a swig of water. What's done is done, and at least my stomach is no longer grumbling.

I make it to the store just in time to take off for the track. Chuck is already there, having knocked back his vanilla latte on the way.

"Hey Cookie," he says.

I roll my eyes begrudgingly. I knew he wasn't going to let it go.

Anyway, what's in a name? Chuck called me "Buddy" during my first time trial. I thought he couldn't remember my name, so he picked a new one. Later I realized Chuck calls everybody "Buddy."

But not me, not anymore. I'm special. For the foreseeable future, I'm Cookie, whether or not I want to be.

CHAPTER FIFTEEN

The Other Side of Heartbreak

AT WORK, ALL writers share the same editor, who in turn oversees several papers. He's unlikely to quibble over the stories we've chosen to report and to write; he's too slammed to propose alternatives.

So when people ask what I write about, I half-jokingly reply that I can write about whatever I want, as long as it's related to Bellevue. Lately, running has been taking up an ever-larger share of my mind space, so I look for ways to write about it (in Bellevue).

This is surprisingly easy to do; runners are everywhere, Bellevue included. Around this time, ultramarathoning has started to take over the running scene; I interview three avid ultramarathoners from—where else, Bellevue.

Every week, in the same space in the paper, there is a feature called "Spotlight." It's a brief profile of someone in the community; that is its only guideline. Often, I'll have a long conversation with the person being featured and boil it down to a few key quotes to feature.

In journalism school, we learned a name for this type of piece: refrigerator-door journalism. It's the kind of trivial content that is meaningful only to the people who are featured in it, and to those individuals, it's precious; worth cutting out and posting on the fridge.

Now that I think about it, refrigerator-door journalism could describe the bulk of these community newspapers. The one I write for is the newest of the papers, and, given the area's rapid growth, also one of the newsiest.

Lately, I've taken to turning the "Spotlight" on local people who do some job in the community, but who I've learned, also happen to be runners. It's an effective trick. People will use the most canned, PR-approved terms to talk about their jobs, companies, and industries, but when you veer into their hobby, they tend to go off script. It seems that no matter how advanced a person is in their chosen profession, if they run, running is the thing they really want to talk about. And when people are really eager to talk about something, they tend to say more interesting things.

One day I get a press release that piques my interest. A longstanding community festival, Seafair, has decided to hold a marathon, which will both start and end in Bellevue. A marathon in Bellevue means I officially get to write about marathon running as news.

I'm sure my co-workers will roll their eyes when they learn of this. Of course, the story will be in the daily paper the company also owns, but rest assured the *Bellevue Reporter* (which is me, basically) will delve into minute details about the race. The course, the people participating in it, the potential economic benefits; I'm going to have plenty of running-related fodder to fill the paper from now until race day.

Also, the chain of newspapers my editor covers has expanded, so there are even more papers for him to supervise. He may not be so thrilled that the *Bellevue Reporter* will temporarily become the *Bellevue Marathon Reporter*, but he's going to be way too busy to stop me. *Success.*

***

UNLIKE MY EDITOR, Coach Chuck always seems to keep himself within earshot of his charges. Always primed to correct an inaccuracy, bust a myth, Coach Chuck can't help himself. Like me, his bullshit detector is always on full blast. I've got the same kind of BS detector, and I know from experience, there's no way to turn it down.

At Chuckit, some of the runners are preparing to run the Boston Marathon. I overhear them discussing the course, and Chuck does, too. Hearing them talk makes me realize I've barely considered the middle miles of the Boston Marathon. My thoughts have to this point focused on what it would be like to achieve the all-important qualifying time and of crossing the finish line on Boylston Street. I know almost nothing about the rest of the course. It still seems like such a lofty dream that I never really stopped to consider the logistics.

I like to think of myself as someone who does her homework, and prepares for the test, who doesn't underestimate things. What a dilettante runner I've been, pursuing a goal with no concept of what it entails.

By the sound of it, the Boston Marathon course is difficult, maybe even as difficult as qualifying for the race seems to be. Only now does it occur to me that the "reward" for running a Boston Qualifying time is, well, running another marathon, an especially difficult one. There is no rest for the weary.

"And then you get to Heartbreak," someone says.

Solemn nods all around.

"Actually," Chuck says. Head swivel in his direction. "Heartbreak isn't called Heartbreak because it's difficult. It's not that steep of a hill."

I look around. These are fighting words. Heartbreak Hill isn't that steep? People are paying attention now. Chuck is about to drop some truth on the fastest, most self-important runners in the group.

"It's called Heartbreak because that's where Johnny Kelley was about to pass Tarzan Brown on his way to win for the second year in a row. And as he did, he tapped Tarzan on his shoulder. But Tarzan responded, pulling away from Johnny, breaking his heart," Chuck explains, a look of contained exasperation on his face, like he's had to explain this too many times.

"That's why they call it Heartbreak."

Chastened and murmuring, runners wander away. If they didn't already know this, no one lets on.

Chuck must've told this story many times, like a teacher repeating curriculum for the current crop of graduating seniors. I'm pretty sure this is the abridged version, so I make a mental note to look it up.

When I Google it later that night, I find that Chuck is right, of course. Not that I ever doubted him. The year was 1936. Although the experience of losing to Tarzan is said to have left him heartbroken, Johnny Kelly evidently got over it. He continued running the Boston Marathon and won it again nearly a decade later, in 1945. He kept on running Boston as long as his legs would let him, completing the race a record sixty-one times.

Tarzan won the Boston Marathon again, too, in 1939. He was a member of the Narragansett tribe from Rhode Island, and his given name was Ellison. (Tarzan initially struck me as possibly a racist nickname, but it is said he was called this by his own people, for his childhood talent for climbing trees and swinging from branches.)

Tarzan didn't just drop Johnny Kelley that day in 1936. Setting out on a record-making pace, Tarzan left him in the dust. The press truck fell behind, following Johnny, who pursued Tarzan for twenty miles. It was assumed that Johnny would pass Tarzan to take the victory again, but after a back-and-forth struggle, Tarzan prevailed.

There are two sides to every story. From the perspective of Johnny Kelley, the final Newton Hill represents heartbreak. But for Tarzan, it was a turning point, the moment that made him a champion. When he finally bested the man who arrogantly tapped him on the shoulder as he passed, Tarzan's heart must've been bursting with pride.

I vow that if I ever have the privilege of running the final Newton Hill, I will remember Tarzan's story at the crest of it. I may be a slow learner, but Chuck's lesson isn't lost on me. We get to choose the stories we tell ourselves. Not everyone gets their heart broken on Heartbreak Hill.

CHAPTER SIXTEEN

Stumbling onto the Front Page

THE DAILY NEWSPAPER has been running some of the stories I've written for the weekly on the front page. This gives me a thrill; it's fun to see my stories grace the pages stacked in newspaper boxes. More people will read and maybe even respond to them.

But it hasn't exactly made me popular with the staff of the daily. I overhear some of them grumbling about it. Why would they begrudge me this success? I'm working for a community weekly. If my refrigerator-door journalism lands on the top of the refrigerator, what's it to them?

I ask around, and eventually, I understand the reason they're unhappy has nothing to do with me or my stories. The problem is structurally based and economic in nature. Most other staff members are in a union, and I'm not—not because I don't want to be, but because the part of the company I work for isn't unionized. Repurposing the work of non-union employees saves the company money. As a reporter for a community newspaper, I'm certainly among the lowest-paid journalists the company employs. I'm the very definition of cheap labor. The daily doesn't have to pay me any extra to reprint my work and doing so saves them money. Journalists vulnerable to cost cutting and layoffs that are ubiquitous in this ailing industry are right to be wary of this tactic.

One reporter pushes back on the repurposing. He doesn't like where it is going. In response, the editor proposes an alternative: He can rewrite for the daily paper the story I wrote for the weekly. It's the perfect corporate manager response, a compromise that antagonizes everybody.

All this time I've been writing harmless, pointless fluff for an audience that I assume barely even bothers to read it. I have been well under the radar of anyone whose opinion matters and finally managing to enjoy the benefits of obscurity. Now, nearly two years into the job, I've stumbled onto the front page. Rather than earning me accolades, it's making me unpopular. I can't win.

It helps to understand none of this is really my fault. The newspaper industry is in a freefall. Our new owners are making some changes, and from the standpoint of the journalists now employed by them, none of them are good. Probably I should be worried about this. And, in the back of my mind, I am. But I still have three more stories to write for next week's edition and also a wedding to plan.

In a few months, Daniel and I are getting married. It's the marriage, not the wedding, that is most exciting to me. We have now been together, in the same city, for two years, or, put another way, throughout the training cycle for three full marathons (Portland 2004, the inaugural Seafair Marathon in Bellevue in 2005, and Portland 2005). Really, though, our relationship spans much more than that, but I don't want to think about all the breakups in the past.

And now, I no longer need to. On August 19, we're restarting the clock. I couldn't be happier.

Morgan comes up from LA to help me plan the wedding. She's an expert planner, so thorough and detail-oriented that friends call her The Morganizer. With me as a bride, she's got her work cut out for her. I've got no budget for this thing, and while I'm thrilled to be marrying Daniel, I've got plenty of ambivalence about the wedding-industrial complex.

And that's just the superficial prenuptial nerves. Deep down, I know it's my dad who's casting a shadow over the planned celebration. When Dan was ready to ask me to marry him, he went to my mom for parental blessing. Like my siblings, I'm much closer to her.

Shortly after my parents' divorce, my dad got remarried. Ever since, he and his wife have had a volatile, tumultuous relationship. It's been a vortex of drama, the kind that can suck you in and pull you under, if you let it.

Determined not to let it, Melissa, Matt, and I have tried to stay out of the fray. Boundaries, the self-help gurus call it. We no longer go to their house, for example. Instead, by his own preference, we always visit Dad at the tavern he's owned since we were babies, often going there together, as a united front. If a wood-paneled dive that reeks of stale beer and grease can be one's happy place, this is his. It even bears his name: Mel's Club Tavern.

Throughout our teen years and now into adulthood, my siblings and I spend holidays and birthdays sitting under the warm glow of a Budweiser sign or stepping over shards of plywood while Dad points out all the "renovations" he has made.

To each other, we raise our eyebrows. It would all be laughable, if it weren't so sad. Nobody is ever going to come to the restaurant he's supposedly going to open next door. Almost nobody ever comes to this bar anymore.

At one time, Dad's existence seemed more comic than tragicomic. Years ago, for example, Dad got through my sister Melissa's simple, traditional church wedding without incident, making everyone laugh. But time spent alone inside this tavern—alone inside his troubled marriage, perhaps—has made him increasingly out of touch with "polite society." Now, if Dad were, for example, to "give" me away in that ritualized relic of the patriarchy, there's no telling what might happen.

So weddings, yay! Daddy-daughter dance, yay!

Even if I actually wanted that kind of stuff—which, for the record, I don't—I highly doubt any of it would turn out well. This is my life we're talking about, not some Julia Roberts movie.

***

EVERYONE HAS TOLD me that planning a wedding is itself a test of endurance, so I hold off on signing up for a marathon. But I am intrigued when I learn that, not far away, a free marathon is going to be held. Immediately, I thought there must be something wrong with it, if it's free. As the saying goes, you get what you pay for. All the marathons I've entered, and every marathon I've heard of, cost one hundred dollars or more.

I email the race director and learn that the Green River Marathon is certified by USATF, which means it is a Boston Qualifier. A Boston Qualifier that costs nothing? I didn't think such a thing was possible.

The race director says he believes it is the world's only free Boston Qualifier, and he intends never to charge an entry fee.

This is contrary to the trends I've been noticing. Other races seem to be adding "runner amenities" and subsequently jacking up their fees. The Rock 'n' Roll Marathon series, for example, has just announced its inaugural Seattle race, and already it's sold out, with people offering to sell their entries for more than the sticker price.

The Green River Marathon seems to be the very opposite of all this. This contrarian approach to marathoning appeals to me, but I'm not ready for another full marathon. I ran my second, the Seafair Marathon, and improved my time by more than ten minutes. In my third, the Vancouver (Canada) Marathon, I acceded to the advice of runners around me—who worried I'd freeze to death in my planned race kit— and wore a long-sleeved shirt under my singlet. Huge mistake. I overheated and finished a disappointing 4:17:02. Never again would anyone tell this Seattle runner how to dress for a race in the rain.

I'm now trying to put that all behind me and build up my mileage again. Low-key and free as an event could be, nobody is going to care if I use the Green River Marathon as a twenty-mile training run. I suggest this approach to some members of Chuckit, and Kris, Corrie, Enid, and I agree to carpool to the start and meet for a buffet brunch at a restaurant near the finish called Salty's once we are all done.

It's early June, with weather that Seattleites call June-uary: cool, drab, and grey, with a heavy overcast cloud cover and unusual humidity. I park my car near a Chevron station in an industrial area of Seattle that I've calculated will be the "finish line" of our twenty-mile run, and we carpool to the start line with a spot on a paved bike path called the Green River Trail.

Kris, Corrie, and Enid all say they've never been here before, but I know this place by heart. For years I rode my bike along this trail, which winds its way along the Green River, around the outside of a shopping mall and retail sprawl, and connects with another bike path that skirts an industrial area and to Seattle.

I can't see any mile markers, but we all have GPS watches strapped to our wrists so we'll know how far we've run. With that, we take off. Within a few miles, Enid and I are running together, with Corrie and Kris somewhere behind.

What I know of Enid I've observed from a distance. We've never run together, and I think she's faster than me. She seems to be a forthright person, serious about her running, and unwilling to suffer fools. In other words, a little intimidating.

But she's not the only one who intimidates me. Several runners are on the course wearing distinctive yellow-and-red shirts identifying them as members of Marathon Maniacs, a newly-formed local group of people so "crazy" about marathons that they run multiple races in rapid succession. The minimum requirement for entry is three marathons in ninety days.

I've been focusing on trying to improve my performance, so to do so many races in such a short span seems like a step in the opposite direction, a vote for quantity over quality.

Enid agrees: What is the point of running a whole bunch of marathons smashed together, without the necessary time between races for recovery and training? Wouldn't it be better to put everything into a single race—whatever the distance—and run as fast as you can?

Marathon Maniacs holds no appeal for either of us. We'd rather run one fast marathon than many slow ones. Our shared belief forms a common bond. It's better to be faster. And while it seems like such an obvious, uncontroversial stance, it is not universal, even in Chuckit. As we enter Tukwila, Enid abruptly brings up a new subject. She's heartbroken, she informs me. The man she'd been dating for several months abruptly ended their relationship. She thought things had been going so well. She thought they had a future. She'd had no inkling anything was wrong when he ended it. Now she's blindsided and confused.

What? Huh?

Enid's sudden revelation hits me like a splash of cold water. We'd been making casual conversation and suddenly she's talking about her love life. Not only is this out of the blue, but it also seems totally out of character for her, at least from what I've observed. At Chuckit, Enid always seems aloof.

How anyone comes to this sort of casual self-revelation is a mystery to me. I've noticed, though, that hours of running seem to strip away people's inhibitions. Things you would never say in polite conversation seem to flow easily when you're a few miles into a run.

I try to imagine the type of guy Enid would date. Already, I can tell, she's intense; for balance, would she go for a laid-back type of guy? She's speaking in generalities, so I can't get a read. Maybe this conversation isn't so intimate, after all.

I've learned that in these situations, the point is not to get to the truth, to get answers, or even to put together a coherent narrative. The facts don't matter because this is about feelings. And the only right answer to feelings are statements that are both universal and affirming. *You'll get through this. It's his loss. It wasn't meant to be.* That's what Enid needs to hear.

Do I believe any of this? I lack the context to know whether they apply specifically to Enid, but the odds are I'm right. We all want to think we're experiencing something completely unique, but all human experience seems to boil down to a few life lessons. In journalism, we say there are no new stories—they just happen to different people. Just because something is a cliché doesn't mean it's not deeply felt.

What I'm feeling is fatigue. We've been running for more than two hours on our point-to-point route, but the conversation is getting circular. I know what it's like to be heartbroken. It's terrible. But my energy, for both running and for listening, is flagging.

Fortunately, there's an aid station up ahead.

Foods I've never seen at a race appear before us: gummy bears, pretzels, potato chips, Oreos. It's like third-graders decided what we should eat. All of it is laid out on a card table, free for the taking. There's also water and Gatorade but no bottles; runners were asked to bring their own, and we have.

I take a handful of gummy bears. Enid grabs a handful of chips. We glance at each other, wide-eyed, as if to say: *Can you believe this is free?* You'd think they were presenting us with a silver tray of caviar and champagne.

Upbeat volunteers staffing the aid station urge us to take some for the road, take as much as we want.

I chuckle to myself.

I'm a woman. In my adult life, have I ever really taken as much junk food as I want? If I took as much as I want I'd be kicking back in one of the beach chairs set up in the parking lot, polishing off the tray of Oreos. Once, I had a cookie before a track workout and got a new nickname for it.

I take as much as I need, which is precisely two Oreos.

We get back on the road, boosted by the sugar rush. Briefly, approaching the aid station, I'd worried Enid wouldn't take any of the food, and I'd feel bad for doing so, but she dug right in alongside me. With fifteen miles behind us, we're now several levels in: I've heard about her heartbreak, and together we raided snacks at the aid station.

There's but one rite of passage left for our burgeoning friendship: our first fight.

The Green River Marathon is a somewhat do-it-yourself affair, so despite copious snacks, we are pretty much on our own when it comes to directions. The course is marked, but the markings blend in with markings made on the pavement for other events, like bike rides. Runners have strung out along the course, and we've got to figure out the way to the end point. We're not going all the way to Alki but instead diverting to the gas station where I've parked my car. I'm going to drive Enid back to hers.

At some point, we've got to figure out where to leave the course, and how to cross over to the other side of the Duwamish River, which cuts through the industrial area south of downtown Seattle.

I take out the directions I've folded up and placed into the pouch with my water bottle. As I understand them, we're supposed to divert off the course nearby and make our way east to East Marginal Way, where my car is parked. If we don't and continue, we'll get hemmed in by the Duwamish River, and there'll be no way to cross back over it. Enid doubts this. She hasn't brought any directions with her, but anyway, she suspects I'm wrong.

It's not that I mind being disagreed with, but Enid never bothered to familiarize herself with the course—as the race advised all runners to do—and now she's second-guessing the plan I've made. She might be right; we might have to go a different way, but she's got no idea which way that is.

A volunteer course marshal is up ahead, directing runners under a concrete underpass.

"Let's ask him," Enid says.

I doubt he'll be able to help us; he doesn't know where my car is parked, but I don't protest. Maybe he can break the stalemate.

The volunteer asks where we're going, and I give him the address of the Chevron station and show him the directions I've printed out. He looks baffled: "Why are you going there?"

"Because that's where her car is parked," Enid snaps. "We're only running twenty miles."

The young man is unable to help us, so we thank him and keep running. Eventually, we encounter three runners who have stopped to check the directions they're carrying with them. Enid explains our predicament to them—my car, Marginal Way, Chevron station—but they can't seem to get past the fact we're not headed for the finish line.

"We're just doing a twenty-mile training run," Enid explains. "We're veteran marathoners."

We're veteran marathoners: her words ring in my head. We aren't earning finisher's medals today, let alone purple hearts. It seems a little over-the-top to say we're veterans, even in the general sense, but I'm pleased Enid counts me in her ranks. I'm a veteran marathoner, just like she is.

Someone finally gives us a ride to Enid's car; she drives me to mine. Once in my car, I check my phone; no messages. Kris and Corrie never passed us, so it's possible they're still on the course. I leave them each a message and head home. No Salty's for me today, I'm salty enough as it is. Corrie and Kris will have to have brunch without us. I hope they're not upset.

This day didn't go at all as I'd planned. I never meant for the group to split up, or to run the whole way with Enid. I thought, in the end, all of us would be celebrating our accomplishment with a brunch buffet.

But that's what happens, I guess, when you're a veteran marathoner. You just go with it.

CHAPTER SEVENTEEN
Nickels and Dimes

FOUR HOURS: IT'S a popular time goal among recreational marathon runners, and it's become a milestone for me. In my first marathon, I wasn't even close, but the result of my second attempt—4:13:07 at the 2005 Seafair Marathon—seems to put me within striking distance.

Progress is not always linear, though. When I overdress for the Canadian rain, and grossly overheat, I take several steps back, finishing the 2006 Vancouver Marathon, my third, in a frustrating 4:17:02. Then, in the fall, I run the Seattle Marathon in a bitter November mix of freezing rain, hail, and ice, and though I'm not overdressed, I nonetheless struggle, finishing in 4:19:49.

I'm confident the conditions, not my training, are to blame. I just need some decent race-day weather, and when I get it, I will take full advantage. On a golden autumn day in 2007, I complete the Portland Marathon, my fifth attempt at the distance, in 3:59:06, so thrilled to have finally run under four hours that you'd think I'd won the thing. I get a little better in the spring, running the Eugene Marathon in 3:57:00. But when I return to Portland in 2008 and run another personal best, 3:55:27, I marvel at how a year can change things.

Running under four hours no longer seems special. Now it's just something I expect from myself.

***

MANY RUNNERS HAVE pre-race rituals. In the past four years, I developed a post-race one. After every half marathon, I go online and plug my finishing time into the McMillan Running calculator, which uses the time to predict performances at different distances. Playing around with the calculator helps me to figure out how far I am from my goal, and what kinds of training paces I need to be able to run to get there.

According to the calculator, based on recent half marathon times, I should be able to run a marathon in 3:53, provided I'm properly trained. This isn't a bad time; it's just not good enough. My Boston Marathon qualifying time is 3:45. I have been inching toward it. But the faster I get, the harder it seems to get faster.

At the urging of my now sister-in-law, Catherine, I sign up for a January marathon in Phoenix, hoping dry weather and a dead-flat course will allow me to improve.

It's the 2009 Arizona Rock 'n' Roll Marathon and marathon number eight for me. The race shirt has a giant guitar on the back. It looks like something you'd find at the Hard Rock Café souvenir shop, not a marathon. Though flat, the course has no shade to shield runners from the blazing desert sun. I do not run well and don't bother to bring the shirt home with me. I'm not going to wear a shirt from a race I'd rather forget.

After training all through the wet Seattle winter, I underachieved again, running the marathon in 3:54, a minute slower than the McMillan Running calculator said I'm capable of. Flying to Phoenix has enabled me to improve my personal best by a whopping forty-seven seconds.

Whoopee.

"You're nickel-and-diming it," Chuck says of my race result.

His words remind me of a conversation that I had a couple of years ago. A woman in the group showed up for track workout wearing a stylish red-and-black jacket from the Boston Marathon, her first. Tall and lean, she is someone likely to be described as "built like a runner," and the jacket fit as if it were made for her.

"I like your jacket," I said.

"It's a great race; you should run it sometime," she curtly replied.

"I'm trying," I said with a sigh, weary from the workout we just completed.

She looked at me intently.

"But are you really, Amy? Are you *really* trying?"

I flashed her an embarrassed half-smile. My face burned bright as her jacket. Best not to answer rhetorical questions, right? Or was it an assertion?

I'd prided myself on making up for what I lacked in running talent with effort and conscientiousness. But she couldn't see it. Or maybe there was nothing to see.

So I began asking myself: *But are you really, Amy? Are you really trying?* The answers were sometimes discouraging. When you lose faith in yourself, or your training, it can feel impossible to get it back.

At the moment, Chuck is coaching more than one hundred people at one time. He can't coach all of us equally or personally, and at times, his generalized instructions to me seem stretched a bit thin.

For example, why do all of us have to run a two-mile time trial once a month, even in months where some of us just ran a race? Stressing out all day and killing myself to get through the bridge traffic to Green Lake so that I can run two miles all out once a month is not my idea of fun. Maybe I'd feel differently about it were I convinced that this effort had a particular training benefit for me, but I'm not so sure about that.

The website with the calculator that I use also has some detailed articles on training. I've been reading them, and I've bought in. I decide to buy a custom training plan from the creator of it, Greg McMillan, for my next big race, the 2010 Eugene Marathon. I'll still be a member of Chuckit, but rather than going along with whatever workout everyone in the group is doing, I'll follow a plan designed for me.

Filling out the questionnaire that will be used to create my plan reveals just how focused I've been on the marathon. I know my marathon PR by heart, of course. It's a new one: 3:51:54 at the 2009 Victoria Marathon, in Canada, my ninth attempt at the distance.

But I've got no idea what my best time is for 800 meters, or a mile, or even a 5K. The question about my weight seems odd, too. Doesn't he also need to know my height, for context? Despite these misgivings, I put down the all-important number, without any subtraction. I figure a coach is like a doctor. If you lie to them, you are just limiting how much they can help you.

About a week after I send in my questionnaire and payment, my twelve-week custom training plan appears in my inbox. I look at the spreadsheet. Some of the workouts, like hill repeats, are familiar. Hills are our friends, Chuck likes to say.

Looks like I'll be making some new friends. Take, for example, the fartlek, a terrible-sounding name for a workout. Fartlek is a Swedish word that translates as "speed play." (So if you're Swedish, running hard is like recess, I guess.) Fartleks consist of several sets of timed hard efforts, with slower and shorter recovery times in between. This fartlek workout is four minutes with three minutes of recovery.

Workouts on the track are also in the spreadsheet, just as I'd feared. I'm not completely over my track anxiety, but it's gotten better. McMillan track workouts take longer to do than the ones that Chuck assigns, so even when I get to Chuckit on time, I'm often left finishing my workout alone.

One evening I'm still running when the field lights turn off. It's after sunset, but there's still plenty of ambient light for me to continue.

"You don't have to wait," I tell Chuck, making a mental note to bring my headlamp next week.

Chuck asks what I'm doing. I tell him: Six to eight times 1,000 meters with 200-meter recovery jog between. Plus three times 200 meters with 200-meter recovery jog. It's as if I'm hearing myself speak a new language fluently for the first time.

Chuck gives me an inscrutable look.

"What?" I say.

He pauses.

Oh, just come out with it.

"That's a lot for you," he says.

If Chuck seems skeptical, my new training plan has Enid intrigued. I sent it to her, and she remarked on the several kinds of workouts that are different from the ones we do at Chuckit. For example, my schedule includes a kind of long run called "fast finish," which is just like it sounds: run most of the run at the usual, easy, long-run pace, then finish the last few miles at the relatively fast race pace, or faster.

One weekend, Enid decides to join me for a twelve-mile fast-finish long run. The plan is to head out for six miles along the shores of Lake Washington, then turn around. When there are three miles to go, we'll speed up, running the final miles at my goal race pace: 8 minutes, 35 seconds per mile.

It's a beautiful spring morning, and the miles seem to fly by, but I have to remind Enid, a former sprinter on the University of Washington track team, to slow it down; it's fast-finish, not fast start. Also, our out-and-back route ends with a few significant hills in the last few miles, which is going to make hitting goal pace even harder.

"Okay, got it," Enid says. At the turn-around point, we make a brief stop to take our energy gels. There is a brisk, early spring breeze. Lake Washington is a deep blue, reflecting the cloudless sky. In the sun, it feels perfect in short sleeves. We down our water and squeeze out the last of our gel packets.

"Get ready," Enid says. "Now for the hard part."

I'm not about to get too worked up yet. We've still got three miles until we need to hit race pace. I glance at my watch as we progress to the final three.

When we're half a mile away, Enid looks in my direction. "Almost there," she says.

"Yep, got it."

Gradually, she is stepping on the gas, so I do, too. Our watches beep three miles to go nearly in unison. Mine says we're already at 8:32, just under goal pace.

"Okay, just hold it here," I say.

Over knotty tree roots that buckle the sidewalk, my steps seem light and quick. A couple of runners coming toward us move to the side so we can pass. This is the first time that's ever happened for me.

We must look like we're on a mission.

"Thanks," Enid says to them, her jaw set.

We are running side-by-side, headed up the steepest of the hills that remain.

"Drive those arms," Enid says.

I'm driving them. I keep driving them.

"Pick up those feet," she commands.

I continue to pick up one foot after the other, as runners do.

We stay steady up the hill; but I'm not going to attack it; doing so would take up too much energy.

And anyway, no need to attack them. Hills are our friends.

When we crest the top, Enid is slightly ahead of me.

"Good job, Amy! Keep it up," she says. "Focus!"

Is she going to do this the whole rest of the way? Doesn't she want to save her breath for running?

My watch beeps, showing an average pace of 8:17, even with the hill. *Wow, that's pretty good.*

A group of four runners is coming toward us now. As soon as she sees them, Enid goes into full-coach mode. She accelerates a bit, widening the small gap between us.

"Focus, Amy! Focus!" she cries. "Drive those arms. Drive!"

The runners ahead scatter as Enid bears down on them. It's a game of chicken, and they lost.

I give them an embarrassed smile as we pass, "driving" and "focusing" like women possessed. But they are too busy chatting to pay much notice.

One mile to go, and Enid knows it.

"Okay, Amy, that's the Boston Marathon finish line right there," she says, throwing her arm to the distance. "Go get it!"

A little ridiculous, but what the heck.

I don't know what our pace is right now, but I'm certain it's faster than it needs to be. Surprisingly, though, it feels, if not easy, at least, inevitable.

Maybe all Enid's yelling is helping. It's entertaining, anyway.

As we approach Madison Park, close to the end point of our run, more people are on the sidewalk, so Enid takes to the street, and I do the same.

"Good form! Good form!" she hollers. "Up on your toes."

A couple walking a pair of fluffy Pomeranians turns to see what the commotion is all about.

You'd think she was training me for the Olympics.

As we come into the final half-mile, I'm running nearly as fast as my legs will carry me. Enid is taking fast-finish quite literally. Glancing for traffic, we flit across the neighborhood's main drag and back onto a quiet residential street, with less than a quarter mile to go.

Somewhere along here my watch is going to beep, and I can stop running.

"All the way, baby! All the way!"

More than the beep of my watch, what I want is for Enid to stop yelling.

Finally, a beep; twelve miles.

Ah, yes!

My heart is still pounding, and I'm breathless, but a glance at my watch showed I was running well under pace, 7:50 on the final stretch. *Not bad!*

Rather than simmer down, Enid yells even louder now.

"That's what I'm talking about!" she hollers, enthusiastically. "Boston Marathon, baby!"

Enid's theatrical coaching makes me cringe like a teenager with a colossally uncool parent. And what's with this weird master-student dynamic? It's as if she wants everyone within earshot to understand that I am the one who is being trained and she's the one giving instruction.

But running so hard and so relatively fast is fun, dramatics notwithstanding. Who knows, maybe the dramatics even help. At least it's a distraction.

After this success, Enid and I start meeting to do our Saturday long runs along Lake Washington, away from Chuckit. Sometimes Enid will run with me; other times her workout is different, so we'll run part together or none of it. In either case, afterward, Enid always goes to the bakery down the block to get a cherry turnover and meets me back in Starbucks, where I'll be swaddled in a sweatshirt, sipping a grande misto in a ceramic cup, extra foam.

Worn-out and exhilarated, we stretch our legs over the extra chairs as if we own them, already nostalgic for the run we just completed. Reflecting on the past week, our training, and new workouts yet to come, the conversation invariably turns to the Boston Marathon. Enid has run the race twice, and she never tires of telling me what a thrilling experience it is.

It's just what I need to hear.

As I flip through the pages of my training plan, I look forward to the long runs that are "fast-finish." Now that I've experienced what it's like to be near the end of a run, yet getting faster and more energetic with each step, I can conjure the feeling, doing it again just by remembering it. I know it's going to be even better the next time.

Lying in bed the night before a fast-finish long run, I feel like a kid on Christmas Eve, so excited about what the next day will bring that I can hardly sleep.

Fast-finish long runs are quickly becoming my favorite run of the week.

CHAPTER EIGHTEEN

Get It in Writing

As soon as I lean back onto the padded table, I realize it's a mistake. My knees lock at a 90-degree angle. I let out a shriek. A member of the medical team tries to massage my legs, but I can't stand to be touched and fear I'll kick him the next time I'm hit with a cramp.

I can't read my watch.

What was my time? What was my time? No one is listening to me. Or maybe I'm not actually speaking?

I sit up, surveying my surroundings, the medical tent of the 2010 Eugene [Oregon] Marathon. So many different scenes of suffering play out before me, it's like a painting by Hieronymus Bosch. Half-naked bodies sprawl on white sheets. One of them writhes in pain. Another slowly rolls over, letting out an anguished moan.

A kindly volunteer removes my running cap, which is soaked with sweat, and hands me a towel. I press my face into it and focus on relaxing my muscles. Someone insists I drink a bottle of water, and some Gatorade, and I dutifully lean forward to get it all down, then put the towel back over my face.

I don't need to be here. The medical tent is a sign something is wrong. And I just had the race of my life, ran 3:44, and qualified for Boston. Wait: Did I?

I take deep breaths, yoga-class breaths. My legs tremble. Out of the corner of one eye, I can see rows of cots full of people much worse off than I am.

The medical volunteer kneads my legs a little more. It's uncomfortable, but I know he's only trying to help. I try not to fight him.

After a few interminable minutes, the cramps subside. Dan must be waiting and wondering about me. He's probably worried. I say I feel okay to go, but the medical staff insists I wait a little longer, drink a little more.

I can't wait to get out of this place.

Someone is moaning again. The cots are nearly full; I should leave.

I did this to myself. What a way to spend a weekend. What a way to spend my life.

I started the race brimming with confidence, determined to follow the plan I'd written in Sharpie on my arm. Whenever it looked like I might be going too fast, I adjusted my speed with a surgeon's precision. But at mile 23, the pace that had for so long seemed too easy suddenly felt impossible.

After crossing the finish line, I went into a stiff-legged walk. My arm extended, I'd been thinking I could support myself on a chain link fence. But my depth perception was off; the fence was well out of reach. My hand dangled in mid-air, grasping for something when nothing was there.

A volunteer came over and put her arm around me. I wanted to keep walking, but she had other ideas. Now here I am among those whose bodies have truly betrayed them. I'm not really one of them, at least.

At last, a medical volunteer finally clears me to go. I make my way out of the tent, through the rest of the finish-line zone cordoned off for runners, and out an opening in a chain-link fence, finally free, back in the land of the living.

A woman rolls out of the tent in a wheelchair.

She just ran a marathon, and now she can no longer even walk.

Suddenly she greets someone she apparently knows with an excited whoop. "I qualified for Boston!" she cries.

I've qualified, too . . . haven't I?

I've lost all track of time; I've got no idea how much time I've spent inside the tent, or whether Dan saw me enter it. But I spot a familiar face, Regina Joyce, a former Olympic marathoner who is now a Chuckit coach, and other runners from the group. Cheerfully, they congratulate me.

What do they know?

Ian, a smiling child psychologist, tells me: "Yes, Amy, you did it."

Well, he's a doctor. He wouldn't lie. But do they know the time I have to run? Are they sure?

Someone tells me I can get a printout of my official time from race organizers. After borrowing a cell phone to call Dan and tell him where to meet me, I hobble to the stand and show my bib number to a volunteer, who prints out what looks like a cash register receipt with the race name and logo and my official finishing time: 3:44:19. The BQ time for a woman my age is 3:45. There it is, in writing: I've qualified for Boston!

It's going to take Dan some time to work his way through the crowd to find me. But the warmth of the sun feels good on my skin. I'm happy to wait here in it for as long as it takes him to get to me. My BQ receipt is safely zipped into my pocket.

In the car on the way home, I get out my phone to text Enid the news. But she already knows; she's been tracking me online. I have a text message from her congratulating me, with several exclamation points. She seems as excited as I am that I've qualified, if that's even possible.

We exchange a few texts. One of them stops me in my tracks: "I think you can run even faster!"

Faster? I just qualified for Boston, with 1:41 to spare, cutting more than seven minutes off of my previous best time. I'm fine with this for now.

This is my tenth marathon. Getting to this point has taken more than five years. In fact, it has taken me so long to qualify for the Boston Marathon that I've aged into a new category, with a slower minimum qualifying time: 3 hours, 45 minutes. Remembering this, I am conflicted. For years I'd set my sights on 3 hours and 40 minutes. But before I could get there, I got older. It's as if someone boosted me over a fence I had nearly climbed on my own.

Now Enid's words feel like a reprieve. She's not suggesting that I'm not fast enough, but that getting even faster is yet a possibility. This means I could run the 3:40 that I set out to run, all those years ago.

Why should this matter? For years, qualifying for Boston has been my finish line. What Enid is saying is that really, it's only the start.

CHAPTER NINETEEN

The Happiest Hour

A FEW HOURS ago, my head was an anvil on top of my body. The pelting rain was heckling me as I tried to finish the Portland Marathon. Somewhere along the course, Lily was doing the same. It was brutal.

Now we are in the bar of our hotel. It was her idea to come here, for happy hour, and it is the best idea either of us has had all day. They don't call it happy hour for nothing.

Lily sighs and takes a sip of her beer.

"Why do we do this to ourselves, Amy?"

The discomfort this marathon has caused us is entirely unnecessary, like extra credit when we'd already aced the test. Lily qualified for Boston a month before I did, at the Napa Valley Marathon, along with Melissa, another runner from the Chuckit group. Chuck had emailed their race times out to the group, and when I saw them, I knew immediately that they'd qualified. It filled me with hope: *I run with them all the time. If they qualified, then so can I.*

On the fourth of July, Lily came over for an Independence Day barbeque that turned into a Boston Marathon qualifying party. Our fellow Chuckit members Kris and Steve brought a Boston crème pie in honor of our achievement. Steve, who had run his first Boston marathon a couple years ago, was especially congratulatory.

"You've really done something special," he said.

Eating Boston crème pie, drinking mojitos, and talking about our plans for Patriot's Day, 2011, Lily and I were on a high. We decided that running a fall marathon, Portland, in October, would be a great way to get in shape for Boston in the spring. It would be marathon number eleven for me.

We were getting greedy, as Chuck would say. Delusions of grandeur, is another way he puts it, sometimes shortening it to "grandeurs," (which sounds to me like a rare type of seizure).

The Portland Marathon was held on the auspicious date of 10/10/10. It was already off to a weird start. That morning, we awoke to a bad omen: a torrential downpour. I felt shaky and congested but thought it could just be nerves. I thought that I could get through it.

Lily had been suffering neck and shoulder pain—the aftereffects of a car accident that gave her whiplash, and recently became dogged by piriformis syndrome, a painful tightening in the muscle deep in the back of the thigh.

It was still dark when we started the race. At the halfway point, I felt super discouraged and I tried to figure out how far it would be to run back to the hotel. But I kept moving, since I didn't want Did Not Finish (DNF) in my results.

I jogged it in at 4:19:09, my black shorts sticking to my thighs like a wet t-shirt contest. When race officials handed me a space blanket at the finish, I needed it for decency as well as warmth. I didn't even want to think about what I looked like from behind.

But I couldn't dwell nor linger too long in the shower; I had a phone call to take. I had just been offered a job as editor of *Real Change*, a newspaper that covers social issues and homelessness and is sold by low-income vendors on the streets of Seattle. I'd been a volunteer freelance writer for *Real Change* for years, completing articles for the paper on nights or weekends and working my regular staff job during the day. When the editor announced his departure, I called him.

"It's the perfect job for somebody," he said.

That somebody was me. I've been offered the job, and now I only have to convince *Real Change* to pay me the same amount I already make.

On this, Lily is my cheerleader.

"You can do it," she says. "Ask for what you are worth."

Lily is in technology sales, a universe apart from the nonprofit sector I am thinking of entering. When I told Lily that I'd have to turn in my iPhone to my current employer and that my prospective one would not be replacing it, she gasped.

"Oh no," Lily said in horror that was only partly ironic, "You can't take that job."

I didn't see how I could turn it down. I knew many in Seattle saw *Real Change* as a "homeless" newspaper, but I understood it as something more: a vehicle for people with resources to engage with people who lacked them, and vice-versa. As editor of *Real Change*, my journalism skills would help build the foundation for any type of social change: relationships. It was hard to imagine I'd be able to have this kind of impact at a job in the mainstream media.

All this is swirling through my foggy brain when I pick up the phone. My hair is still wet from the shower. My legs are aching. But I'm trying to focus on this conversation. Alan, the organization's managing director, is saying something about the Board of Directors, but, I'm so tired, I don't quite catch it.

"I'm sorry. Could you repeat that?"

The salary range, he repeats patiently. It's set by a board of directors. What he just said is so obvious. I can't believe I didn't comprehend it.

I'm extremely low energy, but I don't want him to think I'm just unexcited about the job. On the contrary, I'm very excited. But physically, I'm destroyed.

"Thanks. If I sound a little off it's that I just finished a marathon, and I'm not feeling well, so I'm just not my normal self."

Oh, man. Why did I have to bring up the marathon? Why do I always have to bring up running?

I must be the most annoying job candidate ever, but Alan seems unperturbed. He'll have to discuss my request with the board and get back to me, he says.

I relate this all to Lily, who assures me they won't rescind the offer because I tried to negotiate it in a post-race stupor.

"All you're asking for is what you already make, Amy."

True. But it's the way I asked for it. Why did I have to mention the marathon? He might think I did so in a vain attempt to impress him. Another cringe-worthy moment, courtesy of running.

The waitress informs us that happy hour is almost over, so Lily and I order some appetizers and another round of drinks.

Lily sighs and smiles. I do the same.

None of this really matters, anyway. We raise our glasses in a silent toast, the subject of which is implicit. Despite our weary, bedraggled bodies and my apparent inability not to bungle a salary negotiation, we've both got a reason to be happy. We're registering for Boston next week.

***

I set three alarms for 5:45 a.m. Monday, October 18, 2010, the morning that registration for Boston opens. The application process is conducted online, simultaneously around the world, and race organizers are expecting it to fill up quickly. I debate setting my wake-up time—5:45 a.m., or maybe 5:40—with the intensity and anticipation usually reserved for determining what time to wake up on race day. It feels like a contest. With some 25,000 entries available, and runners all over the world will be vying for a spot in the world's most prestigious road race, not all of us will make it. I'm going to be at the start line when the gun goes off, at 9 a.m. Eastern time.

Anxiety keeps me in a shallow slumber the entire night before, and I resurface at 4:30 a.m., as I have before so many races. An hour later, when the first alarm finally begins to beep, I get up immediately. I'm eager to start the process I fear could take hours.

Also, I'm hungry.

I make oatmeal and brew coffee to fortify myself for what I predict could be a marathon computer session. I sit down at my laptop, with three minutes until the starting gun, click on the registration page just to see if, by some miraculous loophole, the BAA's servers are ready to accept my registration. No dice.

As soon as the clock ticks 6 a.m., I hit refresh, and a blank registration page appears. I fill in the form, check it carefully for errors, and hit send. The form clears, but a new page doesn't appear.

I try again. And again. An hour like this. I take a bathroom break and return. Keep trying. Over and over, I enter the information, auto refill speeding my progress.

I've got to stay positive. I will get in. I check the *Runner's World* message boards on Boston Marathon to see if someone else is having the same problem.

Someone has posted a link to the registration page, so I click on it. It sends me to what looked like the same page I have been using.

I fill it and hit send for what must be the hundredth time.

Miraculously, it works. I am sent to the next page and able to complete my online registration and then given a submission number.

An hour and forty-three minutes have passed, roughly the time it takes me to run a half marathon.

I burst into the bedroom and jump on the bed, where Dan is still sleeping: "I registered for Boston!"

Dan mumbles something unintelligible, rolls over, and smashes a pillow over his head. It's fine. We have months to celebrate. He might as well get some rest.

CHAPTER TWENTY

Safety First

Disappearing into the restroom, I feel like a female version of Clark Kent, or maybe Lois Lane, had she been created in another era. When I emerge, I'm another Amy, swathed in Lycra tights and bright technical fabrics, a headlamp glowing from my forehead, like a cyclops.

As soon as I started as editor of *Real Change*, I put in my vacation request for April 18, 2011. That seems to be the only easy task that I'll accomplish anytime soon. As the interim editor goes over the weekly tasks with me, I feel lightheaded, like I might need to sit down.

I've got to figure out how to fill a twelve-page newspaper each week with a shoe-string staff and volunteers. What seemed from the outside to be a relatively well-oiled machine (as well-oiled as my ancient Jetta, at least) now seems to be held together with figurative duct tape and paperclips.

I can't run away from my new-job nerves, but I can run through them. I need to build up my fitness so, come January, I'll be ready to train for Boston. I have an idea: I'll run home from work. It'll be perfect.

I buy a blue backpack big enough for my cell phone, keys, and, if need be, the dress flats that I wear as work shoes. Everything else I leave to take home on another day. I bring my running gear with me on the bus in the morning, then stash my clothes in my desk to take home later.

I head onto South Main Street, under the crumbling Alaskan Way Viaduct, unsteady on its grey concrete legs, out to the bike path, and into the night. The salty scent of French fries wafts from the McDonald's in the ferry terminal. *Sleepless in Seattle* t-shirts are displayed in souvenir shop windows, referencing a movie almost two decades old, but still iconic here. In the boardwalk-like Fun Center, a carousel sits idle; the horses are stabled for the night. But Red Robin, the hokey chain restaurant that Daniel and I visited on our first date, is still serving up burgers, whose grease I can almost smell as I pass. And here is Ye Olde Curiosity Shoppe, curiouser than ever, hawking the very oddments that as a child I begged my parents to buy for me, including the Mexican jumping bean.

A half-mile away, time nearly catches up with me. The fancy waterfront restaurant where Daniel and I celebrated our second wedding anniversary sits out on the pier, casting reflections onto Elliott Bay. At the sight of this, I get a warm feeling inside.

A few bike commuters whoosh by, but at this hour, other runners are rare. It's dark near the grain elevator, but my headlamp is fully charged, and in my right hand is my reluctant concession to safety: pepper spray.

I keep this with me because one warm evening a couple of summers ago, I was running around Lake Union when a man jumped out of the bushes and began masturbating in front of me. I yelled at him (how I wish I had laughed, or at least stayed calm) and ran across the street and into a restaurant, where I borrowed the phone to call 911. I wasn't hurt, just shocked. I felt like the incident ought to be recorded for public-safety records or something. Because I wasn't in any danger, the operator took my information, and I then finished my run, covering the next four miles at a blistering (for me, anyway) pace.

Amazing what a little adrenaline can do.

About an hour after I got home, a female police officer showed up at my door.

"You were by yourself," she said.

"Yes." I didn't bother to tell her I often run by myself, alone, at night, something dozens of others have intimated that I shouldn't do.

When a string of assaults on female runners (news reports called them joggers, *ugh*) occurred at Green Lake, a city councilmember said women should "buddy up" when they run. You know, because safety first.

Beyond being tone-deaf and sexist, her suggestion struck me as wildly impractical. It's hard enough for women to find the time to train, let alone coordinate our schedules to "buddy up" for each weeknight run.

But this type of advice, coming as it did from an elected official, clarified something: Should anything ever happen to me while running, someone, somewhere will likely blame me for doing something so "risky" as daring to run alone after dark.

So I caved after that incident. I wasn't about to stop running alone at night, so I went to a running store to buy a damn can of pepper spray. The ones in the forefront of the display came in pink, for which they charged extra—typical. I opted for black, the color of my mood.

Now, as I continue toward Smith Cove port, where cruise ships dock in summertime, the canister feels light in my hand. I suspect it might be empty; filled with nothing but false confidence.

The worst part of my run home is here, amid a railyard cordoned off by chain-link fence topped with loops of barbed wire. Streetlights cast eerie triangular shadows over the concrete.

I run up the steep incline and onto a narrow concrete causeway. This is a blind corner; a careless cyclist hurrying home from either direction could mow me down. This stretch makes me think of a prison yard. Whenever I run through it, chain-link on either side of me, barbed wire up above, my pace automatically quickens, and my heart pounds like I just downed a quad-shot espresso.

I tell myself this little jolt is good for me. It gets me out of my shuffling, run-to-commute rut and proves my legs are not as heavy and tired as they seem. *Amazing what a little adrenaline can do.*

A figure hunched under a backpack is making his way toward me on the trail, looking as if he just hopped out of a boxcar.

I'm not afraid of him. He is not the reason I'm carrying pepper spray. I wish I had a way to convey this to him, in the few seconds that will elapse as we pass each other. But I'm not sure it would matter if I could.

And anyway, safety first.

CHAPTER TWENTY-ONE

Let Pain Be Your Guide

I'M NEARLY HOME on my running commute when I feel some soreness in my foot. I decide to take a couple of days off. The Mercer Island Half Marathon is Sunday, and I want to be rested for it.

On the Saturday before, I run for twenty minutes. It's sunny and spring-like and my foot feels fine. We drive to the tiny waterfront village of Hoodsport for a family reunion, for my mother-in-law's side of the family, the Earsleys. To accommodate all who are coming, it's set up in the rural fire hall that Grandma Earsley is responsible for tending; she and her husband have lived in the home across the road for nearly fifty years. Before we're set to start eating, Grandma Earsley asks that we gather in a circle, count off one by one, so that we can see how many are present. Doing so, we see that there are fifty people. After saying grace, and blessing the food, Grandma Earsley has an addition. She notes that Amy is running a half marathon and asks everyone to include me in her prayers.

I didn't expect this, but it's touching. A bit of pressure, too: I feel like I'll be on the start line tomorrow with fifty Earsleys behind me, wondering how I'll do.

My foot begins to hurt at about halfway through the race, a bit past mile 6, impeding my stride somewhat and worrying me. I don't push too hard, and it feels better running uphill and worse down.

Even with the pain, at the finish, I see that I took a minute off my fastest time, finishing in 1:46. After I cross the line, it seems like I have one giant right foot. I loosen my shoelaces and hobble with Enid back to her car, and she drives me to mine.

"Better ice it," Enid says.

When the pain doesn't subside after a few days, I worry. I decide to go to the doctor, then change my mind and decide not to, about 117 times. At work, Alan notices I'm favoring one foot.

"You're limping," he says.

I brush it off. My foot's a little sore from the race, I say. That's an understatement.

After a few days of agony, I make an appointment. On Thursday, I see a doctor who orders an X-ray, a first for me.

The intern waiting in the room with me surmises, reassuringly, that I couldn't be that injured, given that I'd just run a half marathon.

Dr. K breezes into the office, her white coat fluttering behind her like the cape of a superhero.

"Well, you have a stress fracture," she declares. So much for superhero. She seems annoyed, as if I should already know this, and shows me the X-ray on the computer.

A thin line runs across one of my bones, the fifth metatarsal. Metatarsals are long bones in the foot; the fifth one is the one on the outside of the foot.

Dr. K says she is sorry. No running for six to eight weeks.

Um, that's kind of a problem. I'm running the Boston Marathon. When is that? April 18—in twenty-five days.

Dr. K says she's really sorry and offers to write me a note, so I can get my money back on my airfare and hotel. It's as if she is my mom, penning a note to the teacher for my being tardy. I don't think airlines and hotel corporations care much about doctor's notes.

Dr. K isn't getting it. She isn't going to get it, either, so I'm not going to argue. I nod my agreement while crossing my fingers behind my back.

I am running the 2011 Boston Marathon.

At my request, Dr. K gives me a referral to a sports medicine doctor. I walk out to the hospital's reception area and immediately take out my cell phone and dial the number. There isn't an opening until May 8, so I explain my predicament. Boston Marathon, April 18. . . . A sympathetic-sounding man on the other end of the line put me on hold for what seems like an extremely long time.

Dr. Agostini can see me Tuesday.

At home I email Greg McMillan, my coach. He replies with a single line: "Do you have access to an AlterG treadmill in your area?"

I've heard of these before, and I've read about professional marathoners like Deena Kastor and Kara Goucher training on them when injured. I suspect AlterGs aren't cheap. That Greg thinks I, a humble 3:44 marathoner, would even be worthy of stepping on such a high-tech piece of equipment comes as a shock. I figured he would simply suggest pool running or some other type of cross-training.

For someone like me to avail herself of cutting-edge running technology seems wasteful, excessive. When your Volkswagen Beetle breaks down, does the dealer give you a loaner Maserati?

I Google "AlterG" and "Seattle." I find that the Sports Reaction Center, a physical therapy clinic for athletes, has one. Immediately, I email Neil Chasan, PT, the clinic owner.

It's 9 p.m., but Chasan replies within minutes. He cautions me that with a stress fracture, I might not want to run at all, even on an AlterG.

"Let pain be your guide," he says.

**

It SEEMS TO take forever for Tuesday morning to come. At my appointment, Dr. Agostini asks if I can run the half marathon instead. I'm dubious. The Boston Marathon is more than one hundred years old, and it has always been a stand-alone event.

What kind of sports medicine doctor doesn't know this?

I try to answer her questions with patience, even though I don't want questions; I want answers. After a long pause, Dr. Agostini stops pressing on my foot and says I should stop running immediately but that I wouldn't do irreparable harm by running the marathon, although I shouldn't run if the pain goes above a five (on a scale of one to ten).

I am tempted to tell her that for me, running begins at a pain level of five but *WAIT: Did she just clear me to run Boston? Win.*

By the end of the appointment, she has me fitted for an Aircast flexible walking boot, a concrete-colored behemoth that makes me look, from the knee down, like a Star Wars stormtrooper.

When she's done listing the types of cross-training exercises I can do until race day, I ask if I can run on an AlterG.

An AlterG, she repeats, looking surprised. Yes, she says, but she doesn't know any place that has one, except The Human Performance Lab at Stanford's School of Medicine.

Trying not to sound like an insufferable know-it-all (but maybe too late?), I inform her that there's also one at a physical therapy clinic a couple of miles away, one of about 630 publicly available machines across the country.

I leave out the part about having gone to Stanford.

I can try the AlterG, Dr. Agostini says, but "let pain be your guide."

Ah, pain, that fond acquaintance of mine. Marathon running introduced me to pain, and now we are going to Boston together. She will be my guide.

***

A FEW DAYS later, I am digging through Sports Reaction Center's bin of loaner shorts when I remember a quote from Henry David Thoreau: "Beware of any enterprise that requires new clothes."

The shorts, required to use the AlterG, are all form-fitting and long, like cycling shorts. They're unisex and made of something like neoprene, the rubbery wetsuit fabric, with legs so narrow they seem specifically designed for elite Kenyans. The biggest shorts I can find still look tiny. The label says "large." *Great.*

In the changing room, I squeeze myself into the shorts. I'm not sure if it is nerves or my legs being encased in rubber, but I'm already starting to sweat.

The AlterG is visible the moment you walk in Sports Reaction Center. It sits up high, like an altar, behind glass doors in a conference room. The low-end model costs $80,000. I feel like I should genuflect before climbing up onto it.

AlterG stands for alter gravity, and that's precisely what it does. On top of the treadmill belt is a flexible plastic pod that inflates with air, holding the runner up, thereby "removing" a percentage of her body weight. The runner simply punches in the percentage of body weight at which she wants to run. You can adjust this as you run, just as you can change the speed or the incline. In other words, you can "lose" or "gain" weight in real time without even breaking your stride.

I step up and into the pod and zip the apron of the shorts into it. The clinic assistant, Michelle, explains that to calibrate itself, the machine is going to weigh me.

Right now? In front of everybody? Will the machine reveal my weight on its digital readout? Will a robotic voice announce it out loud? They know my shoes are on, right? That's 13.9 ounces per foot!

As the pod balloons up with pressure, it gradually lifts me off my feet, holds me up briefly, and then deflates, ever so gently setting me back down again.

I start out running at 70 percent of my body weight, which AlterG, ever the gentleman, never even mentioned. I can feel anti-gravity working in an instant. My legs feel lighter, my feet do not seem to slap the ground so much as punch it, and they snap back more quickly, increasing the rate they turn over.

If I only I could lose 30 percent of my body weight, running would seem easy.

But it doesn't just seem easier; it is easier. Neil warned me that because the AlterG is shouldering some of the burden as I run, my cardiovascular system isn't working as hard as it would at the same speed on the road. To get the training benefit equivalent to road running, I will have to increase my speed by 7 to 10 percent.

Okay. We'll get to that, in a minute.

I touch the controls on my iPod and scroll through the music. The electronic bleeps and blurps of Simian Mobile Disco flow into my ears. Michelle disappears. I settle into my run. Yes, this is running, and though working out in a darkened conference room in an unremarkable office park, on a space-age machine, is not at all how I'd imagined I'd prepare for Boston, to be training again feels amazing. As for my foot, it doesn't hurt, per se. It just feels weird.

Neil lets me continue for another ten minutes. Then I go to the PT area, where a therapist hands me a clear plastic bag of ice. I recline on a massage table, my upper body swaddled in a towel, the ice melting slowly on my foot, transferring the cold as I transferred my body heat onto the padded vinyl. The therapist sets a timer for fifteen minutes. I flip through a *People* magazine, trying to avoid dripping sweat on the 50 Most Beautiful People.

It hits me that this is part of the workout. Icing is part of my training plan now. I feel pretty legit.

In the morning, I get on the bus to work, my foot encased in the boot, and for the first time ever, I take the elevator to my second-floor office.

The building is old, and the elevator takes an interminably long time going up one flight.

As the door rumbles open, I realize wearing the boot to work is like showing up with a dramatically short haircut. Co-workers are surprised, and some probably wonder how I'm feeling about it. Some may even assume I'm no longer running the marathon. If that's the case, I'm not about to tell them otherwise. I don't know if what I'm attempting is possible, or the right thing to do. I only know I am going to try.

I roll around on my cursed foot, putting it up on a chair whenever I can. I try to act normal. My vacation request was put in even before I'd started this job, and I make no mention of changing it.

To beat the morning commute and still get my run in before work, I try to schedule the earliest AlterG time slot possible. Some days are totally booked; I take what I can get. I drive to Bellevue in my running clothes, sprint-hobble from the parking lot to the building, squeeze into the rubber shorts, and fairly leap onto the treadmill, eager to make the most of my allotted minutes on the machine. My routine would almost be comical if it didn't feel so critical.

One day, I'm particularly excited for the workout to come. I'm wearing, for the first time, the yellow-and-blue running clothes I bought just for Boston. I ordered them online, and a few days later, I came home from work to find a bag from Adidas on my doorstep. I tore into the bag and tried on the clothes immediately, checking out the look in a full-length mirror. Blue and yellow are the signature colors of Boston, and Adidas is the sponsor. I thought that, years from now, I would look at my race pictures and my running gear would look classic, and that I would be reminded of a great day.

But the universe doesn't share my excitement. After practically killing myself to be on time despite the perpetually traffic-clogged bridge that spans Lake Washington, I sit for ten, fifteen minutes into what was supposed to be *my* workout session, watching a bearded young man lope along on the AlterG, headphones on, in the "zone," oblivious to my mental entreaties to Stop. Now.

He doesn't budge.

Wordlessly, I will him to shut it down. He keeps running, as if nothing is the matter. I glance over at Michelle, who flashes a sympathetic, "hang-tight" smile. It's all I can do not to storm into the room, unzip the runner from his inflatable pod, and burst his AlterG bubble.

Time's up, skinny Sasquatch. You are costing me valuable training time that I can never get back.

I remind myself of the saying: A watched pot never boils. I stare at my shoelaces, my cuticles, the carpet, anywhere but at the AlterG.

Finally, the renegade runner stops the treadmill, unzips himself from the machine, and makes a few cursory wipes of sweat from the area.

His red technical t-shirt is soaked. He doesn't meet my gaze. He knows what he's done. The theft of training time is unforgivable. But before he can slink out the door or utter an apology (I know he isn't sorry), I have already stuffed myself into the size-large neoprene shorts and am clambering up onto the AlterG. I've lost enough time; I don't want to waste any more.

CHAPTER TWENTY-TWO

Off the Deep End

NEIL CHASAN IS a former member of South Africa's national rugby team. Stocky and forthright, he looks and sounds the part of cool expat former athlete. The rugby players he works with must love him for it. But part of his business is devoted to runners, which seems to me a decidedly different type of athlete.

But, maybe not.

Chasan comes in to check on me as I'm using the AlterG one day. He says I'm his favorite client because of how happy I look now that I'm able to train.

"You runners," he says, grinning. "You're all addicts."

When I repeat this statement to Daniel, he scoffs. Neil is only flattering me. If I am his favorite, Dan says, it is because by logging as many miles as I can on his bionic running machine, I'm racking up a hefty bill.

It occurs to me I've got no idea what it costs to use the AlterG. Neil never even mentioned it.

I'll probably get an invoice emailed to me. Whatever it is, I'm just going to have to put it on my credit card.

In addition to worrying me, Dan's cynicism stings a bit. Why *wouldn't* I be Neil's favorite client? I might not be the fastest runner that comes into the Sports Reaction Center. (Okay, it's likely I'm the slowest.) But I like to think that what I lack in natural ability I make up for in enthusiasm and commitment. Isn't it possible Neil recognizes this, and it has endeared me to him?

In response to my defensiveness, Dan indulges me with a skeptical smile.

Whatever it may cost, my access to the AlterG is limited. I'm going to have to supplement with cross-training of some sort. I turn to internet chatboards to see how other injured runners manage to do this. Pool running is the favorite, the obvious advantage being that it is essentially the same motion, with less impact. I read a few articles about pool running, and some of them suggest I get a special belt for it.

Beware of any enterprise that requires new clothes. But I want to be prepared to do my "long run" in the pool, so on Friday night Dan and I go to a local sporting goods store, and I buy a Speedo Aqua jogger belt, a rather hideous contraption that I associate with senior citizen women taking water exercise classes.

Look fast, be fast.

The past several years, Saturday mornings have been long-run mornings, a routine I've come to enjoy and to prepare for with ritualized anticipation. Before going to bed on Friday night, I carefully review Weather.com's hour-by-hour forecast and set out an array of running clothes to fit the predicted conditions. At times, this may mean multiple gloves in different thicknesses, sunglasses, hat, and, if necessary, arm warmers. As Seattle Seahawks quarterback Russell Wilson says, "Preparation is the separation."

I also set out my water bottle and any energy packets or other fuel I will need, depending on the distance of the run. If I'm running with others, we often exchange last-minute email or text messages, confirming the location and distance.

That's all moot now. I'm not going outside to run; I'm headed to the indoor pool at my gym. So long, Weather.com! Instead of running clothes I pack a bag with my swimsuit and my brand-new aqua jogging belt.

The fact that I no longer need to complete these little tasks to some might be a relief—once less thing to do—but to me it's a reminder of all I'm missing. The actual running, where the rubber meets the road, is for me the hardest part of marathon training to miss.

In the pool, I can't run every mile as fast as I wish. That's out of my control. But still, it is satisfying to complete all the important things running coaches always emphasize, like being prepared, rehearsing race day, and practicing race pace.

"The will to win is nothing without the will to prepare," Chuck said one day, quoting the great Tanzanian marathoner Juma Ikangaa. The quote pops into my head now.

My preparation now involves finding ways to endure the inevitable boredom of jogging in a small square of water for two hours and twenty minutes. I've chosen this time because it's what it would take me to complete the long run on my schedule.

I rarely run with headphones, but my iPod is a key boredom-beater when I find myself forced to run on the dreadmill. It's not waterproof, though, so instead, I take a portable, battery-operated radio with me and set it on the pool deck. I tune it to a dance-music station and turn it up, the better to hear above the din of the pool area. The acoustics are terrible; the sound is echo-y and distorted, but the good thing about electronic dance music is you can almost always make out the bass.

I jump in the water and click the belt around my waist; properly attired, it is time to get this pool party started. Pool running sounds pretty obvious: run in the pool. Still, as an obsessive, it raises a lot of questions.

Is the belt to hold me up so that my feet don't touch the ground? If this is the case, it seems I need to be in deep water. I consulted the many YouTube videos on pool running but there seemed to be no definitive answer, in large part because all the videos I could find were filmed above the water, making it impossible to see what the pool runner's stride is like and whether their feet touch the ground.

Ugh. Do it right and use a Go-Pro, people. It's not that complicated.

I try out slightly different running positions; they all feel a little weird. Even my normal running motion seems awkward and exaggerated in the water.

How am I supposed to know if I'm doing this right?

The main objective of the long run is simply to build endurance by an extended period of moderate-effort aerobic exercise. It is, first and foremost, a cardiovascular benefit, so I decide to use the metric of "perceived exertion," which is basically noting on a scale of one to ten how hard you feel like you're working.

It seems to be much harder to get my heart rate up in the pool. The resistance of the water makes pool running feel anaerobic, like pushing a giant rock. The graduated depth of the pool means one end is too

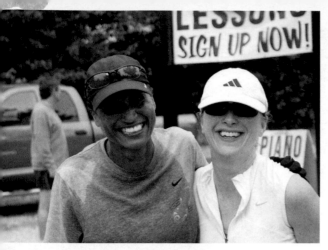

Enid and I take a break at an aid station in the 2009 Green River Marathon. We ran twenty miles of the free, low-key race as a training run. *Photo by Steve Hamling.*

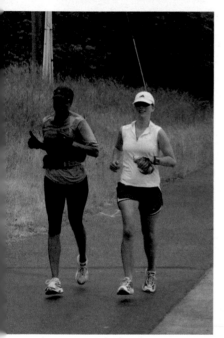

LEFT: The event ended up being the first of many long runs that Enid and I would do together. *Photo by Steve Hamling.*

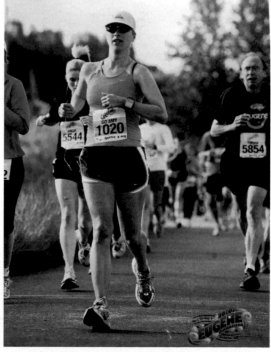

In the early miles of the 2010 ugene Marathon, where I qualified for the Boston Marathon for the first time, I tried to stay calm and focused.

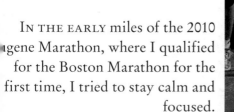

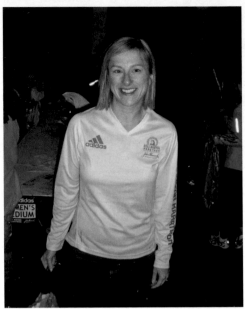

LEFT: Although I tried on the 2011 Boston Marathon Finisher shirt for size as soon as I got it, I didn't wear it until after the race; I didn't want to jinx it. *Photo by Daniel Liberator.*

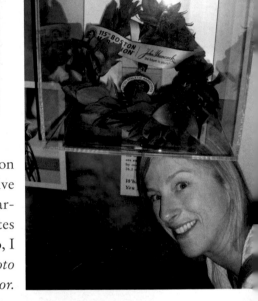

RIGHT: The winner of the Boston Marathon is crowned with an olive wreath made from branches harvested in Greece. This tradition dates from 1984, and at the 2011 Expo, I attempted to "try on" a replica. *Photo by Daniel Liberator.*

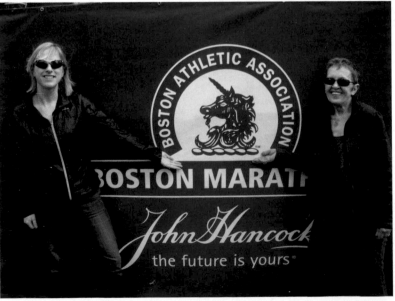

My mom traveled to Boston for my first Boston Marathon, and here she shares my pre-race excitement. *Photo by Daniel Liberator.*

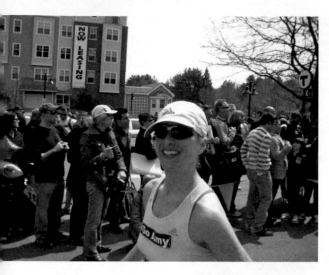

"IT'S THE RACE of your life," Daniel said as he ran alongside me to take this photo during my first Boston Marathon, in 2011. *Photo by Daniel Liberator.*

LILY AND I were so both so thrilled to have finished the 2011 Boston Marathon that we randomly posed in front of Ann Taylor Loft. *Photo by Daniel Liberator.*

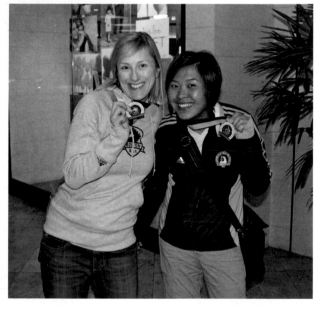

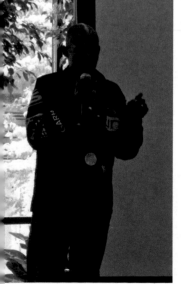

AS HE SPOKE to runners before the 2012 Eugene Marathon, Meb Keflezighi proudly showed off the silver medal he earned in the Marathon in the 2000 Olympics in Athens. *Photo by Amy Roe.*

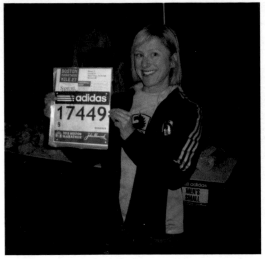

How low can you go? Low bib numbers are generally associated with faster qualifying times. Here I am with my second-lowest bib number to date, in 2013. *Photo by Daniel Liberator.*

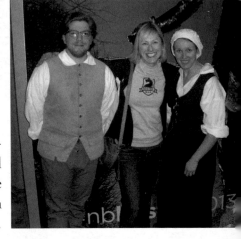

People dressed in Revolutionary War-era garb were on hand as part of a Paul Revere-themed campaign New Balance created in celebration of the 2013 Boston Marathon. *Photo by Daniel Liberator.*

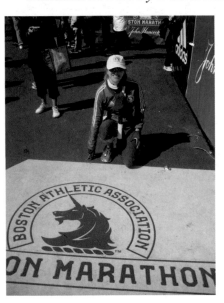

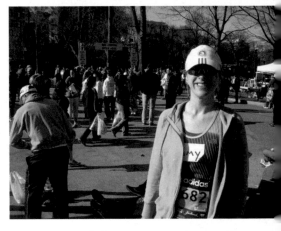

Thousands of runners flock to the Boston Marathon finish line for a photo like this one, from 2014. Many are careful not to cross it—they save that for Patriot's Day. *Photo by Daniel Liberator.*

It's my third time at Boston, but I've still got "first-day-of-school" nerves as I prepare to board the bus to the start line in 2014. *Photo by Daniel Liberator.*

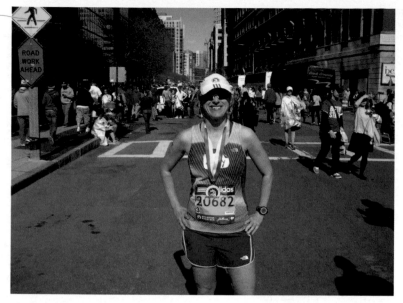

THE 2014 BOSTON Marathon felt like no race I've ever run, and after finishing I was even more jubilant because of Meb Keflezighi's victory. *Photo by Daniel Liberator.*

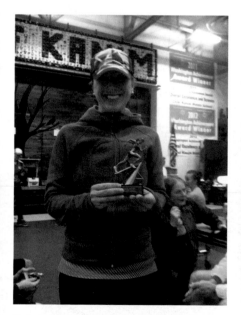

IT'S NEVER TOO late to be a contender. I got the first sports trophy of my life when I placed third overall at the 2015 Fall City 10K. *Photo by Daniel Liberator.*

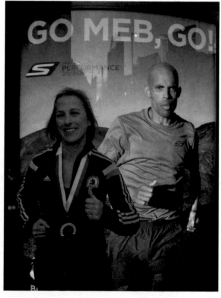

ON THE WAY to the 2014 post-race party at Fenway Park, I couldn't resist the opportunity to be pictured "running with" Meb, the first American Boston champion since 1985. *Photo by Daniel Liberator.*

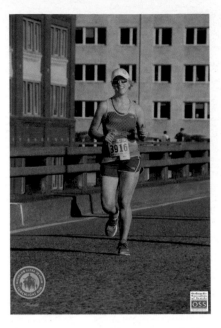

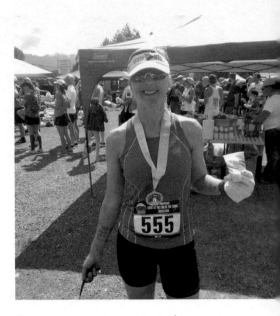

As my running progressed, I began racing shorter distances, and enjoying them. Here I am in the 2014 Seafair Torchlight Run 5K in Seattle.

Referring to splits written on my arm helped me stay on pace during the 2017 Light at the End of the Tunnel Marathon where I clocked my fastest time: 3:37:25. *Photo by Daniel Liberator.*

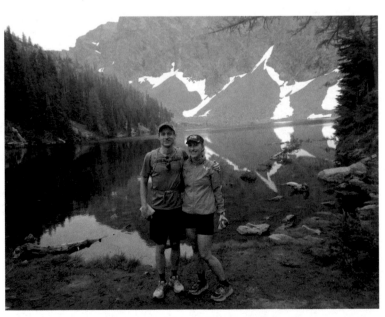

Although he's not a marathoner, Daniel often does short runs with me. Here we are on a trail run in the North Cascades in 2017. *Photo courtesy the author.*

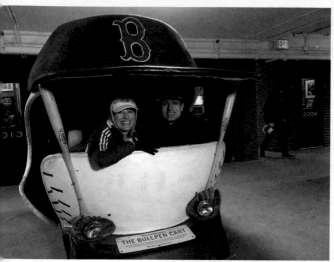

THE TEMPERATURE WAS in the thirties and it was snowing when Daniel and I attended a Red Sox game the day before the 2018 Boston Marathon. We warmed up inside this bullpen cart. *Photo courtesy of the author.*

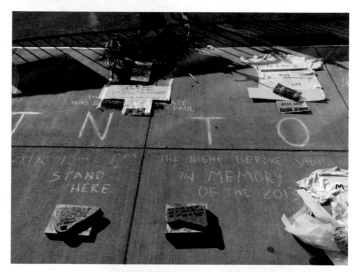

RUNNERS RETURNING to the Boston Marathon in 2018 honored those lost and injured by placing mementoes at the site of the 2013 explosions. *Photo by Amy Roe.*

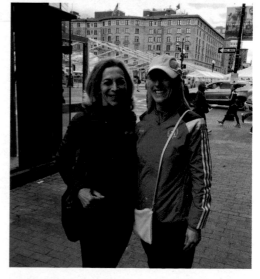

..TING BOSTON MARATHON trailblazer ..athrine Switzer the day after the 2018 ..n Marathon was a lucky coincidence. ..inded me to stand up straight for this picture. *Photo by Daniel Liberator.*

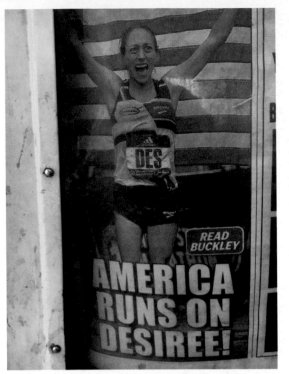

Des Linden was on the front page of newspapers across America on April 17, 2018. This *Boston Herald* headline, with it Dunkin' Donuts reference, was my favorite. *Photo by Amy Roe*

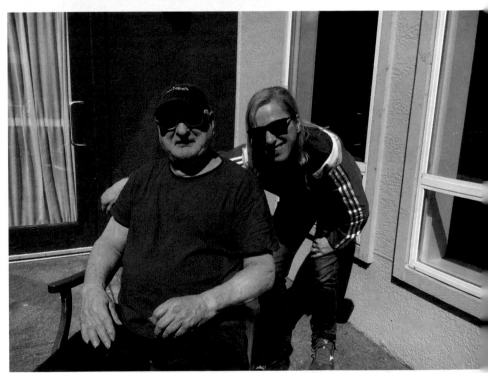

I was disappointed with my performance in the 2018 Boston Marathon, bu I still wore my jacket to visit my dad afterward. *Photo by Daniel Liberator.*

shallow for me to run in, so all that's left is the deep part of the lane I'm in.

Run the mile you're in.

To jog back and forth feels more normal and interesting than staying in place, so I make partial "laps" up and down the deep end of one lane, which, fortunately, I have to myself.

Swimmers enter the neighboring lanes, complete their laps, and leave. Next to them, I feel like a hamster frantically turning its wheel, doomed to stay in the same place no matter how hard I exert myself.

The tinny sound of the radio gets louder and softer as I complete my "laps" of a quarter of the pool lane. Sometimes a forceful kick or stroke from a swimmer in an adjacent lane sends a wave in my direction, momentarily carrying me down the lane like a leaf in the wind.

It takes all my concentration to maintain my rate of exertion and long-run effort. When my mind drifts, I find myself slowing down, bobbing leisurely, rather than propelling myself purposefully. A giant swim clock mounted on the wall ticks away the seconds and minutes. When I was on my high school swim team, we used a clock just like it to time intervals, the second hand relentlessly pushing us through the workouts. Now it helps me time my water jogging "laps" and ensure I maintain some semblance of long-run effort.

The many cross-training articles I'd read about water running talked about how effective runners have found it. None of them mentioned the mind-numbing monotony. I'd always said I love being in and around the water. Who would've thought being trapped in a humid, loud, chemical-smelling room, doomed to repeat a mundane activity until it is burned into your nervous system, would be excruciatingly boring?

I hate the treadmill, but at least there is the sensation of speed, a satisfying thwack of feet pounding the belt, and the gratification of "miles" or "pace" tallied up in a red digital readout.

Still, this wet, smelly hell isn't for nothing. I think back to the message-board posts from injured runners who describe in excruciating detail their extensive cross-training regimens, some of which produced surprisingly good results on race day. Especially encouraging to me was an account by a woman who'd spent hours on an elliptical machine when she couldn't run and found herself not far off her personal best when she eventually completed a marathon. Other marathoners recounted completing grueling stationary cycling sessions or back-to-back spin classes that enabled them to be remarkably prepared on race day. Even healthy marathoners are known to submit themselves to heroic acts of tedium. A friend of mine, confined to a basement treadmill by severe weather, completed multiple twenty-mile runs on it, without even so much as a window to gaze out of as she did.

This is just what it takes.

The radio falls silent; the battery has died. It needs to be either recharged or plugged into an outlet, but I can't do either. I didn't bring the adapter with me to the gym.

A gym employee walks in. Standing at the far end of the pool, she trains her eyes carefully at me, hand on her hip, as if I'm in for a scolding. Someone must have told her that a lady had been jogging in the pool for an unusually long time. Is she giving me the side-eye, or is this just due diligence?

I just smile and nod. *Nothing to see here.* Luckily, after a few minutes, she leaves.

For all my planning, it hadn't occurred to me that I might run out of battery power.

So now it's just me, and the pool, and the sound of the water lapping into the pool filter and being sucked out, like the tide flowing in and out of a coastal grotto. I listen closely, the better to hear the faint sound of the gym's in-house soundtrack (complete with commercials) on the other side of the clear glass window that separates the pool from the weight room. But I can't hear the music.

So I sing to myself under my breath: Pop songs, inspirational power-rock anthems, I spend monotonous minutes mentally scrolling through my iPod and trying to remember a playlist. When I don't know the lyrics, I make some up.

This passes the time surprisingly well. Just when you think you can no longer take it, something changes, and you feel as if you could go forever. And the best part is that it is preparing me for Boston.

CHAPTER TWENTY-THREE
Fragile Mammals

WHEN I SAW the hairline fracture on the X-ray on my foot, it was confirmation that what I feel was real; my mind wasn't playing tricks on me. Now, my mind is always focused on that fifth metatarsal. I will it to heal, and when I step down on my foot and felt the ache this creates, it seems I'm breaking it even further.

How does a bone heal? Do the cells grow together?

I picture a hard, white stick, the handle of a porcelain teacup. I concentrate my mental energy on the bone. I try to heal it, like an illusionist, with my mind.

Somewhere I read that horses and humans are the only animals that get stress fractures. This makes me think of Tinkerbelle, an Italian greyhound who pranced into our lives a couple of years ago. She was the featured animal in a "Pet of the Week" program at my work. I was instantly smitten by this sweet, watchful little creature. Daniel and I were familiar with the breed and knew they were affectionate little dogs who didn't require a lot of space—a perfect choice for apartment dwellers like us. We'd be talking about adopting a dog for a couple of years. Immediately, I left early and went to the Humane Society, bringing Tinkerbelle home with me.

It's surprising to think this little dog, with her long, narrow femur, so fine that in bright sunlight it is nearly transparent, is nonetheless not at risk for a stress fracture. Surely, I'm not more fragile than this little creature. She must be more vulnerable than I am. But despite her delicate bone structure, Tinkerbelle is immune to the injury that has befallen me. Among mammals, I am the weakest kind.

Some articles I've read online suggest supplements might contribute to healing, since calcium is important for maintaining bone health and density. At the grocery store, I get a value-sized canister of chocolate-flavored calcium chews.

I love chocolate, but I'm kind of picky about it—a chocolate snob, you might say. As part of an effort to improve my nutrition during training, I've cut back on my usual daily consumption of dark chocolate; you know, the healthy kind.

But the calcium chews, though made with high-fructose corn syrup, can't rightly be called candy. Individually wrapped in purple foil, the squares look like fancy little caramels but taste like Nesquik turned into taffy. The container says they have five calories per piece and two have 100 percent of the daily calcium requirement.

This isn't chocolate, it's medicine. Medicine meant to heal my fractured bone.

I find myself dosing two or three times a day, immediately balling up the foil wrappers and throwing them away, so as not to end up with a pocketful of "evidence," as with Hershey's Kisses people set out in bowls at Christmas. This leaves me no reminders of just how many chews I've chewed. All I know is I'm burning through the massive canister and eager to replace it.

Despite what I'm telling myself, I'm developing a taste for these sticky little morsels. They are filling a void. The anxiety of not being able to train for Boston has reduced me, pathetically, to an addiction to calcium chews.

In an injury-induced slump, I've also developed another vice. The internet is a seemingly infinite compendium of free and untested advice, a substance nearly as addictive to an injured runner as calcium chews. Runners who have struggled with stress fractures post lengthy, detailed recovery tips on running forums and blogs. Most say to limit my walking, which jibes with what my doctor has advised.

I make walking-avoidance a sport of its own, going to great lengths to get off my feet and stay there. At work, I roll around on my desk chair, dragging the bulky plastic Aircast with me like a ball and chain. I vow to eliminate nonessential brick-and-mortar shopping, and at the grocery store, I make use of one of the electric mobility scooters parked "for guest comfort and convenience" at the entrance. Motoring through the narrow aisles of the supermarket, I attract a few quizzical looks, but I pretend not to notice.

My fellow shoppers go out of their way to be helpful, offering to get things for me from high shelves. I'd rather they ignore me entirely, but I try to be appreciative and nonchalant, all the while feeling guilty and faux-gracious.

"It's just a stress fracture," I say, trying to deflect the attention. But this seems to make people feel even sorrier for me.

"Oh, dear," an elderly woman replies. "That sounds painful."

Lady, you have no idea.

***

SINCE MY INJURY, Enid and I haven't been able to run together, though we've emailed and talked on the phone. The weekend before the race we meet for brunch at a café near the University of Washington that's known for its fruit bar, where you can heap piles of fresh, organic berries on whatever you order for breakfast. I stand in line on the crowded sidewalk. My boot is in full view as Enid drives up. She knows I'm in a boot, but even so, when she sees me she stops her car in the middle of the street. I brace myself for her reaction. Enid can be loud and dramatic, even in the best of circumstances.

"Oh, my GOD," she exclaims through her open car window. People on the sidewalk turn to look. I wave her over to a parking spot and go to check on our table.

Maybe it helps that I'm wearing the boot because my name seems to come up quickly on the waitress's waitlist.

As we sit down at our table, I see another friend, Erica, seated with her family across the room. But she doesn't see me. My boot secret is safely hidden under the table, out of view.

I order French toast, and it comes with a dollop of whipped butter that melts slowly, sending a white rivulet around the plate. It's delicious, but I don't feel I'd "earned" it with a run, and I don't want to gain weight during what has become an abrupt taper for the race.

Enid, who is in the middle of intense training for a half marathon in which she hopes to PR and win her age group, digs in. We review her training and goals for her upcoming race. We talk about Boston, and again she recounts her two experiences there, and how thrilling they were for her.

Regardless of what is going on inside the gray boot I'm wearing, it's nice to spend time with someone who thinks of my running Boston as a good thing. A few non-running acquaintances have implied running the marathon is a risky decision. At least Enid understands.

"I'd crawl that race on my hands and knees," she says, and I'm pretty sure she's not exaggerating.

As I return from the restroom, Erica catches my eye from across the room and gives me a "What the fuck?" expression. I smile and rock over to her table.

"Oh my God! The marathon!" she says.

"I'm still running Boston," I said, trying to sound casual and unafraid. "It's not as bad as it looks."

That's not entirely true. I don't know how bad my stress fracture is. It must look worse than it feels. Is this a white lie, or maybe a blue-and-yellow one?

Enid and I clean our plates, and she asks the waitress to take our picture with Enid's phone, for posterity, and probably, for Facebook. It's the last brunch before Boston, but by the way Enid is talking—and the way we have eaten—you'd think it was The Last Supper.

"This is it," she says, portentously. And the camera snaps.

CHAPTER TWENTY-FOUR
Break a Leg

WITH A BOOT on my foot, I've become painfully observant of something: Stairs are everywhere; up from the street to our apartment, and inside of it; on and off the bus; and to the office where I work. *How did I never notice this before?*

The boot makes stairs slow and difficult, but I'm supposed to wear it whenever I'm outside of my apartment. It's cumbersome, but I've only got a few weeks until Boston. The boot is helping me get there.

I'm making my way down the stairs to the sidewalk, one step at a time, Tinkerbelle's leash in one hand; the other hand is on the rickety wooden railing.

I can see my neighbor Carla down on the street, a look of concern on her face.

"What happened?" she asks. Standing above her on the stairway, my boot is on full display.

After I finally make way across the street, I explain my stress fracture, the Boston Marathon, and all the hoops that I've been jumping through to make sure that I get there. Carla nods knowingly, swinging her long blonde hair to one side. Carla lives next door, and since Dan and I have lived here, she's been somewhat of a mythical neighborhood creature: a ballerina for Pacific Northwest Ballet.

Carla has an adorable toy fox terrier, Bella, who is smaller than Tinkerbelle, and interested in being her friend. Tinkerbelle is skittish about this, a dynamic that always makes us laugh and forms the basis of my interactions with Carla thus far.

We never exchange more than friendly tidbits—the type of things that you would talk about with any acquaintance. She's mentioned when going back to Brazil in the summer to visit family; or when she's rehearsing a big show, and we've made small talk about our dogs. But never before has Carla inquired about my life. Now she knows about Boston and everything that it encompasses for me.

Dancers get stress fractures all the time, she says. I'm not surprised to hear this. I know from all the dance movies I've seen that dancers are masochists. Like runners, I guess.

"Call me this weekend," Carla offers. "I'll show you how to tape your foot."

She gives me her cell phone number, and I tap it into my phone. I feel a little flutter. *I have Carla's cell phone number. We've both got tiny dogs; we've both experienced stress fractures. Me and this glamorous ballerina, we're practically BFFs.*

I count down the days until I can call Carla.

Does she really mean it? Will I get to see her place? What do professional ballerinas keep in their condos?

On Saturday, after returning from my two-hour pool run, I dial Carla's number, and just as I'd hoped, she answers right away. "Sure, come on over," she says.

What do you wear to a professional ballerina's home so you don't look fat?

I take my most flattering jeans back out of the laundry basket and throw on a sweatshirt that's more like a stylish athleisure top.

Carla's condo is spotless and silent. She is in dancer-casual wear just like in the movies: leggings and cashmere socks and a long, close-fitting knit top. Outside, walking Bella, Carla is always bundled up in a chic coat.

Now I can see how lean and perfectly muscled she is. She looks like she does Pilates in her sleep.

In my jeans and sweatshirt, my limbs are several times the circumference of Carla's. If you bundled three Carlas together, I'd still be bigger. But of course; she's a professional dancer. I'm a professional at, um, writing. I could diagram sentences in my sleep. But my plies leave a lot to be desired.

"I'll go get the tape," Carla says, and disappears up a long stairway.

Her home is built like mine, tall and narrow. But of course, it's taller, with vaulted ceilings and three stories instead of two. The windows are large. It's overcast but lots of natural light streams in through them.

While she's gone, I glance over at Carla's open kitchen. There is a basket of fruit and some containers on the counter, probably filled with quinoa or other ancient grains. Carla must eat only whole foods. I imagine she does a lot of cooking. Probably, she's gluten-free and vegan. I bet she never has a cookie from Starbucks before rehearsal. I bet she doesn't eat cookies at all.

Carla returns with several rolls of tape in different colors and a binder. We sit on the floor with them, on a soft woolen rug covering the gleaming hardwood floor. Carla mentions that her partner, John, is a "healer" who does "body work," by which she obviously means the human, not automotive, kind.

I have seen a much older man entering and exiting Carla's condo. So that's John, her partner. It's a pretty convenient set-up, if you ask me.

Carla asks what I do for work. I'm a reporter, I say. Online news. Oh, so you pay a lot of attention to the news, she asks? Yes, I answer, and Dan does, too. (I guess I want to show her that my partner also compliments my work habits?) We both work in the media, at the same company. We talk about news all the time.

I don't love the sound of these words, but they are not untrue. I wonder if Carla is the type of person who only reads the *New York Times*, a true sophisticate who is not especially concerned with local news, and its special elections, and school board meetings, and property tax levies. But she seems interested now, or at least she's polite enough to act like it.

It's possible that her rarefied world doesn't allow for much news at all. Carla could be on a low-information diet. She doesn't consume any junk food for the body or mind. Why gorge on garbage when you're making art?

Flipping through the binder, Carla shows me the various types of taping one can do. We discuss the RICE (rest, ice, compression, elevation) protocol, often used to treat injuries.

I explain what the doctor told me; she confirms this with her experience. I won't hurt myself further by running on my foot, she says. Dancers perform for years on stress fractures. They just take a lot of Advil, she adds, matter-of-factly.

This is both appalling and intuitive. If you are a professional dancer at a major company like Pacific Northwest Ballet, there's always someone waiting in the wings, ready to take your place, an understudy. Your sick day could be their big break. The pressure to perform, and never be sick or injured, must be intense.

Also, I note she says Advil, and not the generic name for the drug, Ibuprofen. Maybe professional dancers can afford brand-name over-the-counter drugs. Or probably, it's just given to them for free at work, buckets of Advil for the taking, like donuts in the break room. Advil should sponsor a dance company, get their name on the program—the PNB, powered by Advil.

Unspooling the tape, Carla begins wrapping my foot to support it, then gently crisscrosses around the toe. The tape is pliable and surprisingly comfortable. She pulls it tight against my foot, my calloused, unmanicured toes sticking out from underneath.

The tape is blue. It reminds me of the track, the teal shorts I followed through my first Chuckit time trial.

"Blue is a calming color," I say. This is a corny thing that I would never normally utter aloud, but here in Carla's townhouse, something's come over me. I'm a different Amy; more spiritual, more organic. I'm taking on her vibe.

"Yes," Carla agrees. "Each of the colors of the tape correspond with an energy. The energy is healing. This is what John's work is all about."

Now I'm in over my head, enthusing about healing energy, even as mentally, I'm mocking it. But it *is* as if I can feel the blue tape healing me, or maybe that's just what I *want* to feel. Blue helped me get through my first track workout, which at the time seemed like an insurmountable obstacle. Maybe blue tape can help my foot heal, too. John's healing abilities may have rubbed off on Carla, and she is healing my stress fracture this very second.

I would like to believe this. But I also know that there's probably no science behind it. All of this sounds like pseudoscience to me, or at least, the placebo effect in full force.

It has been said a mark of intelligence is the ability to hold two opposing ideas in one's mind at the same time. Maybe I'm not as intelligent as I thought, because I really can't take this holistic energy thing seriously.

I want to be more like Carla, an artist, dancer, dreamer, believer. But I am a journalist, skeptic, realist, pragmatist.

I need to find a way to be all of these, at least for the next few weeks.

CHAPTER TWENTY-FIVE
Boston with Swagger

I AM SITTING on a bus, going to work, when Dr. Agostini calls, right on schedule, for our "phone visit." She asks me how it is going. *How the hell am I supposed to know?* The boot is a huge encumbrance, and whether my foot is healing inside of it, I have no idea, and in one week, I'm going to try to run 26.2 miles on it.

But Dr. Agostini sounds so gentle and concerned I don't say any of this.

"Okay, I guess."

I ask Dr. Agostini if I can take off the boot and try running, just to test it out, before I leave for Boston.

I can run for ten minutes or so, she says hesitantly, but I have to "let pain be my guide." *Bingo. I've got permission.*

The next day, I'm at the track at Seattle Pacific University, a few blocks from home, wondering if pain will show up today. I walked here, slowly, feeling exposed to be outside in running clothes, and without the huge boot on my foot.

Strides have been part of my training for years now. You run the long side of the track and jog the ovals. It's a chance to practice good running form, and to do a little bit of faster running, with quicker feet. But I've never really been able to wrap my head around what my running form is or how to improve it, so I concentrate on the last part: quick feet.

The track is rubber, soft and bouncy, the color of a basketball, but the real reason this facility was built is the soccer field it surrounds. The track was clearly an afterthought. There isn't enough room for a full

oval, so it cuts inside, narrowing in strange angles. It's hardly regula-
tion, but I've gotten used to it. It isn't awkward; it's special.

I haven't run on the ground for weeks, and it feels like I've forgotten
how to. My ankles are brushing up against each other, as if I'm holding
my legs too close together. Every few steps, part of one leg inexplicably
comes into contact with the other. It feels wonky.

I do two laps, a tiny fraction of a marathon, running the straightaway and jogging the curve. I've got 26.2 miles of pavement ahead of me
and two legs that won't stop bickering.

"How'd it go?' Dan says when I walk through the door.

I don't want to say I might have to run an entire race wobbly as a
newborn fawn, the Bambi of the Boston Marathon.

"Okay, I guess. My foot doesn't hurt; it just feels weird."

"Weird how?"

I explain the ankles-hitting-each-other thing. Like I've lost a bit of
motor control.

"That *is* weird," Dan agrees.

***

DAN, MOM, AND I are waiting in line to board a red-eye to Boston when
I overhear a woman ahead of me say that she's run seven marathons. I
recognize the track jacket she's wearing. It's a blue and yellow Adidas
jacket with the words "Boston Marathon Qualifier" printed where a
breast pocket would be.

I'm holding the boot in my hand in front of me. I'm not going to
wear it around, but I'm taking it with me just in case my foot starts
hurting, and I need to rest it.

The woman in the jacket turns to me and asks if I'm running the
marathon.

"That's the plan," I say with a tentative smile and a nod at my boot.

She says she's injured, too, and plans to walk the race.

Her injury must be bad, if she's already made up her mind to walk.
Now it is decided: I have run several more marathons than she has, and
I'm not walking this one.

After landing in Boston, we all need breakfast. A hotel worker
directs us to a nearby diner. I haven't been to a real diner since the last

time that I was on the East Coast, and I'm ready to make up for lost time. I order a chocolate chip waffle and scrambled eggs with Swiss cheese. Even my mom, ever the discerning Seattleite, is satisfied by the strength of the coffee. It's good.

A group of women enters the diner, each of them wearing the green-and-black 2011 Boston Marathon jacket. I thought there was some sort of taboo against wearing the jacket before having finished the race, but all around us are people in green-and-black gear emblazoned with the words "2011 Boston Marathon." Some people are even wearing the yellow 2011 Boston Marathon finisher shirts that came in the race packets.

I'm glad to see people reveling in their hard work and good fortune to be running the marathon. It adds to the festive atmosphere. However, I'm refraining from wearing any such regalia until the race is safely behind me. There is the matter of my foot, but mostly, it's that I've waited this long—I can wait a few more days.

When I turn in my card to get my race number, I ask the volunteer if I can keep it as a souvenir. I feel a bizarre attachment to every scrap of paper with the BAA logo on it. But the volunteer says no; she needs to keep the card as proof that I picked up my number. This kind of accounting keeps people from running under someone else's name, she explains.

I get it. It's important to maintain the integrity of race results. And there are plenty of souvenirs for sale and for free just a few hundred yards away, inside the race expo.

I've heard that Boston's Expo is one of the largest in marathoning. It certainly seems bigger than any I've ever experienced. The cavernous, windowless exhibition space inside the Hynes Convention Center is buzzing with the low roar of thousands of people talking, probably about their race goals. It's so vast that race organizers included a detailed map in our race packets.

I use the map to plot my plan of attack. First, I secure the prized Adidas poster several people have told me about. This year's version says, "Boston With Swagger."

Swagger? I'm hoping not to limp.

At the John Hancock booth, I collect another coveted freebie, the BAA/John Hancock "26.2" sticker. Most other races have 26.2 stickers, but I never felt the need to have one until I saw the blue-and-white

Boston Marathon version. I've got no plans to put this on my car, but I take a couple anyway, including one for Enid. The two times she ran the Boston Marathon, the stickers were not yet a thing. This year, the Boston Marathon has much better marketing.

Among the many exhibitor tables, I spot a familiar brand: Kinesio tape, the kind Carla used on my foot. I explain my stress fracture to a Kinesio tape rep, and she offers to tape it up for me, just like Carla did.

But do they have blue tape? I ask, half-jokingly.

"Oh, sorry, we didn't bring any blue," the rep says, sounding sincerely apologetic.

I sit down, take off my shoe and sock, and present my foot to a Kinesio tape specialist, who painstakingly weaves two colors of tape (green and black—to match this year's Celebration jacket) around my foot in an elaborate pattern designed, she says, to stabilize the muscles in my foot, relieving pressure on the bone I'm trying to heal.

My foot feels good, swaddled in the contrasting colors. But I'm not exactly crafty. How will I ever recreate her intricate handiwork, I ask.

You don't need to, she says. You can keep this same tape through Monday. Just don't get it too wet, and it should be fine.

I don't even need to buy any tape? I'm good to go as I am?

Yes, the rep says. Have a great race.

I hurry across the convention center on my newly reinforced foot. It's time to get in line to see Ryan Hall. At the time, Ryan is the American record-holder in the half marathon and believed to be among the strongest Americans in the elite field this year. He finished third in 2009 and fourth in 2010. He is looking for his first win in 2011.

When the line moves far enough that I can spot the top of his shaggy blonde head, I realize Ryan is sitting down, saving his legs. He's wearing jeans and running shoes by Asics, his sponsor. His face is lean, and his skin stretches over his prominent cheekbones, taut as a drum.

To me, Ryan looks ready. But what do I know? When it's my turn, I present my poster to him and tell him it's my first Boston Marathon.

He tells me it's his third. I know this but don't say so. I just smile, and he smiles, too, because what comes next is obvious.

"Third time's a charm," Ryan says.

As he signs my poster with a Bible verse and a loopy John Hancock, I mention that I also went to Stanford. It was grad school, I wasn't an athlete, and anyway, I've read interviews where Ryan said he'd struggled at Stanford, trained too hard, had issues. But it's the only connection I can think of, and in the brief time we have together, I'm going to use it.

Ryan grins again. He came down from altitude to do a few of his final training runs near the Stanford campus, he says, nodding his head like a California surfer dude.

"Good running mojo," he says.

***

EVER SINCE WE landed, I've known this moment was coming. It's the shakeout run. I've got a lot to shake out.

Dan and I walk out of the hotel and head toward Boston Common, all kitted out in running gear for a jog that's going to take all of ten minutes. Runners from all over the world are here, speaking excitedly in many languages. I'm struck by how small most of them are, tiny people.

Were they all born this way, or have they been winnowed by their training?

I'm comparatively sturdy, a corn-fed American. My size-ten running shoes seem enormous; any bigger, my Dad used to joke, and I'd have to wear the box.

A street is closed, and people are striding back and forth on them like it's a drag-racing strip. It's not where I'd planned for us to run, but whatever. I look at Dan; here it goes.

I click my watch, and we start jogging gently. We make our way down the block and loop around it; another street is closed, plenty of room to run.

My foot feels . . . not good. Maybe it's just not warmed up?

The air is fresh and cool; it's overcast, with a few late-afternoon breaks in the clouds. The trees are blooming and so are the flowers. I inhale deeply and try to relax. My body knows what to do. And I am here, in Boston for the marathon.

Finally, after all this time! It is beautiful.

The path along the Charles River is nearby, and I'd love to run on it, but it's farther than we're running today. My foot is officially throbbing now.

What. The. Fuck.

We return to where we started, and I stop my watch. Dan doesn't ask how my foot is, and I don't offer it up. He knows.

"Maybe I'll ice it tonight," I say, knowing I will do no such thing.

In fact, when I go back to the room and find the Kinesio tape is peeling, I rip it all off.

I don't need Kinesio tape. I can only imagine the blisters it would give me. I never trained with it, so to enter the race with it would be to defy the golden rule of marathoning: Nothing new on race day.

Lily, the running buddy from Chuckit with whom I just ran the Portland Marathon, picked the restaurant where we're meeting her and her boyfriend, Andrew, for our pre-race dinner. It's not far from the hotel and exactly the type of place I would've chosen myself: a modern minimalist space done up in white; a menu of carb-heavy Italian food that's neither too bland nor too spicy.

I order a pre-dinner cocktail because, oh, what the hell. It's not like I'm running for time tomorrow. Mom, Daniel, Lily, Andrew, and I make a toast, as we're celebrating early. Not too early, I hope.

Lily lists all the gear she bought at the expo. Andrew smiles.

"She worked so hard to get here," he says. "She might as well."

Dan glances in my direction. He teased me about my purchases; three running caps emblazoned with the official unicorn logo (in the Seattle rain, I often run in a cap) one of the jackets everyone is wearing, a sweatshirt, and running tights.

As I unpack all of it in our room, showing each piece to my mom, Dan raises an eyebrow. Compared to Lily, I showed restraint.

"I guess you could've bought more stuff," he murmurs.

***

IN THE MORNING, Dan walks me over to the Boston Common, where Lily is waiting, cup of coffee in hand. The forecast is cool and bright, excellent marathon weather.

This is it!

Dan takes our picture, and Lily and I get on the yellow school bus to Hopkinton with our plastic gear-check bags, much like it's the first day of school. The bus driver wishes us luck as we head out the door to the Athlete's Village.

I'm going to need it.

The giant, inflatable arch at the entrance marks the Athlete's Village. Lily and I stop to get our pictures in front of it, like kids with Mickey Mouse at Disneyland.

Inside, we find our fellow Chuckit runners—Melissa, Bill, and Seanna, who've claimed a spot of grass on the ground next to a tent where bagels, Gatorade, and water are available. The sun is warm, but the breeze is chilly.

The wait inside the Athletes' Village is supposed to be long. I'm wearing a sweatshirt I bought at Goodwill so I can throw it away, and I'm glad it's heavy. Everybody has told me it will feel like forever before it's our time to line up. And maybe it feels long, in bad weather, or by yourself. But, huddled in the sun, distracted by our chatting, time flies by. Melissa notices people with blue bibs are leaving; the announcer called our group to the start already.

The race is timed by chips embedded in each race bib, so technically, your race "clock" starts whenever you do, but I hadn't planned to saunter over and hop in on a whim.

Our wave, the blue wave, has been going to the corrals for a while now. We've gotta get going.

On our way there, a race photographer stops us for a photo. We pull up our sweatshirts to show off our bib numbers and smile. This is it. We made it!

After dropping off our gear-check bags in the window of a school bus, we file down a lane created by white picket fences. People are lined up alongside the fences, some of them clapping and cheering. We haven't even started the marathon yet and already there's applause.

I wave at the spectators, my hand in white manicure gloves I borrowed from Mom when I realized I didn't bring any, and it was going to be breezy. With them on, I feel like a princess in a royal procession.

The corrals we are supposed to have waited in no longer exist; the volunteers tell us we can just go up and run over the start line whenever we want. It all feels like a letdown. No announcements, no national anthem. Of all days to show up late for something.

I look at Lily and Melissa, a few steps in front of me. I need to get my GPS watch ready. Wait up, what's happening, guys?

Melissa has the fastest qualifying time of the three of us, and no injuries to slow her down. Comfortingly, like me, Lily is not 100 percent; her neck and shoulders are stiff and pinched, the aftereffects of a fender bender this summer that left her with whiplash. The three of us cross the timing mats as if we're just out for a long run. I hit start on my watch as I cross the second one, knowing this is goodbye. We've no plans to run together. We're on our own now, in a crowd of thousands.

Adidas has set up banners on the course marking the cities on the route.

"Hopkinton With Excitement," the first one says. The course starts on a downhill, so mile 1 flies by, in 8 minutes and 47 seconds. Hopkinton with a little too much excitement.

An aid station has been set up just after mile 2. It's arranged exactly as Enid had said it would be, with water and Gatorade on either side of the road, eliminating the need for runners to crisscross the course. I'm not thirsty, but I grab a water cup anyway, take a few sips, and, with a fluid, practiced motion, toss it aside. Taking water at each stop in the early miles is a tactic I use to regulate my pace. Rather than focus on running, I concentrate on being a smooth water-taker, spilling nothing, sipping easily, chucking the cup clear of the course with a decisive flick of the wrist. It takes only a few extra seconds to do this, which is perfect because in the beginning of a race, I'm usually moving a few seconds too fast.

Another blue banner is strung over the course: "Ashland with Stride." My strides are nothing like the ones I did on the track before the race. My legs haven't brushed against each other once. I'm running normally. Nice and easy, mile 3 in 8:51.

I'm running the Boston Marathon!

The route is less rural now, with more development. "Framingham with Confidence," a banner near mile 5 declares. I'm confident too. It's still early, but my foot doesn't hurt.

A man is yelling at runners up ahead. He's pointing to a building behind him along the course. I don't understand what he's saying, but I remember a book I read while I was training that describes each mile of the course in minute detail. I realize he's gesturing at the furniture store with mirrored windows where you can see yourself running the Boston Marathon.

Just in time, I get a glimpse of my yellow tank top and blue shorts reflected in the window of the store. I wave, my white glove flashing in the mirror.

It's really me; running the Boston Marathon, in Framingham, with confidence, at least for the moment.

Somewhere up ahead of me, the elite runners must still be racing. I wonder how the top Americans—Ryan Hall, Desiree Linden, and Kara Goucher—are doing, and whether they're getting the benefit of the tail-wind everyone has been talking about.

It seems like we've entered the Boston suburbs now. Commercial buildings line the road, which dips down and passes over a blue-grey lake. We head into the center of town, and my surroundings are New England-y again. At mile 10, we're in the historic part of Natick, or as the Adidas banner puts it, "Natick with Nerve." Crowds of people line the course. Children hold out their hands for high fives. Their parents smile and wave. I've cut off the top of a personalized race bib and pinned it to my shirt.

"Go Amy," it says, and people are taking the hint. "Go Amy!"

I'm still taking my water every mile. I strip off my gloves and toss them aside. The sun is higher and bright; my hands are getting hot. But we've all got something to look forward to; Wellesley is next.

Much to the chagrin of people who, in bad weather years, have assumed there is an actual tunnel where you can get out of the elements, the Wellesley Scream Tunnel is a metaphor, not an actual tunnel. Nonetheless, it is legendary; it's the first part of the Boston Marathon course I ever heard anyone mention. Wellesley College, which admits only women, was founded twenty-two years before the Boston Marathon, and students have cheered on every running of the race. After the BAA began allowing women to enter as official participants, in the 1970s, the tradition of cheering runners on took special significance. It's been said that that's when the screaming really started. When the elite women run by, the fervor of the Wellesley women reaches a fever pitch.

People say you can hear the screams from up to a mile away. All I can hear are the pounding of feet around me, breathing, and the rustle of the breeze.

How close are we?

The course is tilting downhill now, but slightly. I'm nearly halfway through the Boston Marathon and my foot feels . . . fine? A little weird? But I know by now that in practice, 13.1 miles is not halfway in the marathon. The race really starts at mile 20. There's so much running left, maybe it's best not to think about it.

The area is wooded, and smells fresh, like evergreens. It's a bit like we're back in the country now. I listen: Is that it?

It is. A blue banner introduces it: "Wellesley with Screams." All the runners around me seem to quicken their stride. Up ahead barricades line the road, bodies pressed up against them.

As we reach the barriers, the sound is deafening. I've heard people can unconsciously surge on this part of the course. I remind myself to slow down and take it all in. Almost all the young women are holding signs, dozens of signs, in all manner of markers and tagboard. Most of them start with "Kiss me."

"Kiss me I'm an economics major," "Kiss me I'm from Florida," "Kiss me I'm Single," "Kiss me I'm an Equestrian."

Kiss me, I've got a stress fracture.

The Scream Tunnel stretches out for 600 meters, at least. I'm on the right side of the road. Wellesley women spot the "Go Amy" on my shirt and yell. "Amy, Go Amy!"

The women of Wellesley are cheering for *me*.

"Woo, Amy! Come on, Amy!"

I pick up the pace, then remember to slow it down. A bunch of college women are screaming their hearts out for me. Why not just enjoy it?

Despite my intention to savor it, the Scream Tunnel fades to a murmur in a matter of minutes. I'm sorry it's over, but up ahead, runners appear to be perking up. We are approaching the halfway point in the race. A camera has been set up above the course, capturing images of runners from overhead.

I look up at the camera and give a double thumbs-up sign. So far, so good.

At the next part of the course, somewhere in Newton, a sprawling, affluent Boston suburb, I see her. Mom's red hair makes her easy to pick out of a crowd. Also, she is literally jumping up and down when she recognizes me. She waves her arms wildly and hollers. Dan runs alongside me, trying to snap a photo. I slow down so he can get it.

"It's the race of your life," he says, eyes wide. I'm touched by how much he wants me to enjoy this experience and not feel anxious about my foot.

I'm trying. At the moment, it's working.

The course is undulating now, these must be the Newton Hills I read so much about. A banner confirms it: "Newton with Grit."

But I can feel myself slowing. I remember being a pace leader: even efforts, not even splits.

Some people are slowing to a walk, the hill is getting steep. I concentrate on the pavement just in front of me and on moving my feet quickly.

I'm not walking, at least. How will I know when I am at the final hill, Heartbreak? It doesn't matter. As the saying goes, run the mile you're in.

Heartbreak must've happened somewhere back there, because the course is descending, and I can see the Prudential Center in the distance and then a fluttering blue banner, "Brookline with Ambition."

It seems to be getting louder with each step. The crowds are crazier; I feel like I'm running on the sidelines in the Superbowl Stadium.

"Go Amy," people shout, little kids and their moms, teenagers, even, see the black words on my yellow shirt and scream.

I am looking for a sign: the Citgo Sign in Kenmore Square. When you can see it, you are two miles away from the finish. When you run under it, you've got just one mile to go.

Instead, I spot the blue Adidas banner. The biggest one of them all, it stretches across the side of a building.

"Boston with love," it says.

The finish line must be just up ahead of me. I might be able to duck under the four-hour mark. It's a reason to push harder, and I do.

The screaming, cheering, excitement on the faces of strangers: I missed all of this the first time I saw the Boston Marathon years ago. It has existed only in my imagination ever since. Today I'm a part of it.

Right on Hereford, left on Boylston; t-shirts at the expo contained nothing but these words, a reference to the street signs ahead of me. I'm entering the turn on Boylston. It's so loud, tears begin to well up in my eyes. But I've heard other runners say you can't run and cry; you need to be able to breathe. I inhale, turn the corner, and let it all out: Portland Fit and Chuckit, hill repeats, the Wall of Death, calcium chews, AlterG and taping, getting fired and getting hired, getting married, giving away books, track workouts, long runs, the McMillan running calculator, chafing, sweating, running with Lily and Enid, running alone. All of it has brought me here, to the Boston Marathon finish line, in 4:03:07. Boston with swagger; Boston with love.

The next day, I'm back in the boot again, rocking with Mom and Daniel through the Isabella Stewart Gardner Museum, extremely grateful that in the grand old mansion where Isabella used to live, there are now ramps for wheelchair users.

"Did you finish?" a smiling man asks me, seeing my boot. People have been asking me this all day, congratulating me heartily when I say yes.

After all my worries about the stress fracture, it's my toenail that forced me back in the boot. During the race, I developed a blister underneath it. My toenail now sits atop the blister like a high hat, and the entire toe is bruised black. It's swollen and tender, disgusting to look at. But fortunately, it's the same foot as my stress fracture. I put the boot back on to protect it. Out of sight, out of mind.

About the time I was thrilling to the scene at Wellesley, history was being made in Boston. It turns out there *was* a tailwind. Geoffrey Mutai of Kenya finished in a course record of 2:03:02, the fastest time a man has ever covered 26.2 miles. (Mutai's performance was not considered a world record because Boston, a point-to-point course with significant elevation drop, is not eligible for world records.)

So fast was the race pace that the top four men all came in under the course record, including Ryan Hall.

Ryan ran from the front during much of the race, and Geoffrey credited him for setting the pace early, pushing Mutai to what is now being called a world best. Ryan's fourth-place finish, in 2:04:58, was the fastest marathon ever run by an American.

Some questioned Ryan's front-running strategy, but in interviews, he seemed utterly satisfied with his performance, referring to himself as a "2:04 guy."

Good running mojo, indeed.

The women's race was equally exciting. Desiree Linden, whom I just missed getting to see at the expo, battled Kenyan Sharon Cherop down

Boylston Street for second place, and lost to her by two seconds, the closest finish in Boston Marathon history. Her finishing time, 2:22:38, was the fastest ever run by an American woman at Boston.

Despite how well she'd run, Des described her performance as a letdown. She had for months thought of herself as the winner. Crossing the finish line that day, though, she wasn't.

As I enter the most notorious room in the Gardner Museum, Des comes to mind.

In 1990, the Museum was hit by the largest art heist in history. Thieves stole 500 million dollars' worth of art, thirteen paintings in all, including two paintings by Dutch Masters Vermeer and Rembrandt. The frames that used to surround the paintings still hang on the wall.

It's jarring to see them, two rectangles of wood with nothing but wallpaper inside. I imagine that's kind of how Des must've felt yesterday, with everything set up perfectly in her mind; and then the real-life image is missing.

But the masterpieces may yet be returned to the museum. And Des, too, may have her day.

CHAPTER TWENTY-SIX
The Robo Rabbit

ONE MORNING IN 2010, I saw that Kris had sent me a link to a website.

"I don't know when this starts, but this is not good," she said in her email.

I clicked on the link, which brought me to an official-looking statement on "mybaa.org" that the Boston Marathon would be adjusting its qualifying times.

"What? OMG are you kidding me? WTF?!" I replied to Kris.

And then, I did what I should've done in the first place. I Googled it. It was an April Fool's Day prank.

Duh.

The site even said this, in tiny print. But I should have recognized it by the fake web address. "Mybaa.org" is not the web address I've so often visited over the years.

I emailed Kris back.

It's a joke, I said. Stand down, everyone. All of us on the email chain agreed it wasn't funny. It did turn out to be a harbinger, though.

The 2011 Boston Marathon field filled in an unprecedented eight hours, sixty-five times faster than the previous year, one newspaper reported. Lily and I were among the lucky ones. About three thousand runners who had qualified tried to enter but were shut out.

This prompted the BAA to make some changes to its registration process and to tighten the qualifying standards for the first time since the 1980s. I'd worked for so long to qualify, and now that I was into Boston, I felt the ground shifting under my feet.

The new standard for me would be 3:40, the qualifying time for me when I started this whole marathon running business, in 2004 at age thirty-one.

Would my Boston Marathon finisher's medal now mean less because it was achieved under the "old" standard?

It was a reminder I never met the time goal I'd set all those years ago. It was a reminder of the feeling of having been boosted over the fence that I'd nearly climbed on my own.

After I calmed down, I tried to find an upside. After I finished the Eugene Marathon, Enid said she believed I could run even faster. And now, the BAA has given me my reason to keep trying to do so.

I'd worried that, like a greyhound chasing a lure and having finally caught it, I would see that the rabbit was mechanical, and thus lose the drive to chase it again. The Boston Marathon race organizers rebuilt the rabbit, making it a kind of robo-rabbit, a Terminator rabbit that can perhaps never be caught.

Perversely, this makes me want to try.

Two years after the April's Fools Day joke that no one laughed at, I'm returning to the Eugene Marathon. It's 2012, and I'm a different runner now. In my bag I've packed my Boston Marathon jacket as well as my Boston Marathon hat (as part of my race day ensemble) and a New Balance Boston Marathon t-shirt, should it get too warm for the jacket. Obviously, I'm determined to make a statement.

Enid and I joke that I must wear the Boston jacket to the expo under any conditions—even if it is so warm out I have to wear a tank top under it.

"In the club, baby," she says.

Just a few years ago, I would've mocked such behavior as cheesy and self-congratulatory. It probably is. Part of me would like to be the type of person who doesn't need to signal to others that I am "in the club," who runs for the purity and beauty of running itself, oblivious to status symbols.

But I'm not that person yet, and looking around the expo, I'm in good company. Boston Marathon jackets are everywhere. Eugene, home to the University of Oregon and its legendary track teams, bills itself as "Tracktown USA," having been home to dozens of legendary runners over the years. Further, it is the birthplace of Nike, and in 2007, it got a namesake marathon.

Among the featured speakers at the expo is Meb Keflezighi, winner of the 2009 New York Marathon and silver medalist in the marathon at the 2004 Olympics in Athens. These highlights alone make for a remarkable career, but what's equally impressive is how well Meb has performed throughout his long career. He was the 10,000 meters champion in the 2000 and 2004 Olympic trials and once held the USA record in the 10,000 meters. His numerous podium finishes at the New York Marathon date back to 2004, and at Boston, he's placed third (2006) and fifth (2010).

Everybody loves a winner, but not everyone wants to hang out with one. Meb is different; relatable. So many people have shown up to see him speak that it's standing room only. We end up way in the back.

Lily lent me his book, *Run to Overcome*, in which Meb describes leaving his native Eritrea as a child and finally settling with his family in San Diego, where he discovered his talent for running.

Much of what Meb is saying now at the Expo seems related to his book. This must be his typical stump speech, but it is especially compelling to hear it in his voice, rather than the one in my head.

"Okay, I've got a little surprise for you all today," Meb says. He unzips his track jacket and pulls out a silver medal hanging around his neck. It's from the Olympic Marathon in Athens. The real deal.

Despite our distance, I have no trouble seeing the look on Meb's face. He is grinning so broadly it's as if he won that medal yesterday.

Dan glances over at me, and we both smile.

"Pretty cool," I whisper. He knows what I mean: Cool that he won an Olympic medal, yes, but cooler still that, eight years later, the thrill Meb gets showing it to others is palpable, even here in the cheap seats.

Back at the hotel, I stop by the front desk to request a late checkout when I hear a voice from behind me.

"Oh, you can run a marathon faster than that."

I turn around and see a man of about thirty smiling at me. It is true I've run a marathon with much more time to spare, but I want to be able to take my time showering and cleaning up after the race.

I don't say this, I just smile, and give him a wave.

A couple hours later, I see him again in the lobby. He's using the microwave to sterilize baby bottles.

"How did Boston go?" he says. I tell him the race was fantastic, but I don't elaborate, but because I sense his question is only a prelude, and it is. He's here to qualify, and he tells me all about it, reeling off his running resume, including his PRs at various distances and the brand-name races he's run. He flew to Eugene from Houston, Texas, where he lives, for the race. He just missed qualifying at the Houston Marathon, a few weeks ago.

Eugene is a good race for a BQ; I earned my qualifying time here in 2010, and I am back to do it again, I say, trying to project confidence. I *am* confident. I don't mention the new qualifying standard I'm trying to hit, because this is not about me, really. In my magical jacket, I'm playing the role of the Boston Marathon fairy godmother, spreading lucky pixie dust among the hopeful.

He looks down at the floor, and, never meeting my gaze, reels off a list of close shaves that almost got him his qualifying time, and what he'd run where and when and under what conditions. If I didn't know better, I might take this as symptoms of a mild form of autism.

But it's only nerves. How much he has invested in qualifying, how much it would mean to him if he did—these are things few people anywhere understand, and he knows I am one of them.

If only I had a way to turn his tentativeness into confidence. If only this jacket were magic.

"Good luck," he calls after me, as I walk toward the elevator.

"See you in Boston," I say.

***

THE NIGHT BEFORE every race, members of Chuckit perform the pre-race ritual called making a Little Chuck. This involves laying out every item you will wear in the race, including your race bib, carefully pinned in advance, as if dressing a scarecrow. Some people take a picture of their Little Chuck and post it on Facebook.

I've always chosen what I wear on race day carefully, sometimes weeks in advance, as part of my preparation. Look fast, be fast. Enid believes bright colors are the way to do this. This is no time for some tattered old race shirt. You want to look pro, not, as Enid puts it, "hoe-dee-doe."

"Slammin!" Enid says when I show her what I'm planning to wear. It's a bold look for me and reveals a new level confidence. I'll be wearing a tank top in radiant hot pink, a shade that Adidas calls "ultra pop." My shorts are steel grey with pink, coral, and white stripes down the side, in a classic style Adidas created in a tribute to legendary Norwegian marathoner Grete Waitz. The first woman to run a marathon under 2 hours and 30 minutes, the world record at the time, Waitz took silver to Joan Benoit's gold in the marathon at the 1984 Olympics in Los Angeles.

All of this—the bright colors, the association with Grete—I count them in my corner. But my most powerful asset is the excitement I feel. My training was imperfect. It was interrupted by a nasty cold that sapped my energy and filled my head and chest with fluid. There was my badly botched half marathon and the fact that I had not set any PRs in my build-up to Eugene.

All of this is outweighed by the fact that I am entering this race having completed a dozen marathons, including the 115th running of the Boston Marathon, a notable day because it was the day that a world-best men's marathon time was made. I'll be wearing a Boston Marathon running cap from the 2011 race.

I've done this before; I can do it again.

In the morning, I pop right out of bed, having slept little. I shower and put on my sunscreen and running clothes. I eat my plain bagel in the lobby area, so as not to disturb Dan, who tends to sleep right up until ten minutes before we need to leave. It never bothers me; I know he'll get up when he needs to, and I like the quiet time alone.

When I get to the start line, I hear a familiar voice. The announcer has handed the mic over to Meb, who is serving as the race's official starter.

This is the day you've been working for, Meb says. You've told everybody at work, and you know when you go back to work they're going to ask how your race went.

People chuckle at this.

Meb reminds us to "run to win," which is one of his sayings. Nearly every one of us has zero chance at coming in first, but I know what he means. For some people, winning may be just getting to the start.

I think of the runner I met in the hotel lobby yesterday. I never got his name.

Good luck, dude from Houston. I hope you make it.

CHAPTER TWENTY-SEVEN
Takes One to Know One

THIN AND PALE, with a black knit cap pulled low over his ears, Nick shows up at my office looking more like a juvenile on work release rather than a college student on winter break.

It's January 2014, and Nick has applied for a reporting internship at the nonprofit weekly newspaper where I work. His resume notes he was a standout runner in high school and is now attending a Midwest liberal arts college on an athletic scholarship.

I've already made up my mind not to bring up running with Nick. It's not relevant to the internship, and I don't want it to give him an unfair advantage over others. But my opportunity to avoid it soon disappears.

"I see that you ran the Boston Marathon," Nick says, his face blank, his voice flat.

Obviously, Nick has Googled me and is thus familiar not just with my professional resume but my running one as well. It's good for a reporter to do research. To be the subject of it is discomfiting.

I try to sound friendly and nonchalant. I explain that I ran the Boston Marathon first in 2011 and then again in 2013 and given the "events that occurred at the finish line," I am going back in April for a "do-over." I am trying, perhaps too hard, not to make the whole thing sound fraught with emotion.

Nick doesn't say a word. I can see sweat marks forming on the armpits of his shirt as he sits there, staring at the floor.

I change the subject. Nick hardly needs to ingratiate himself to me by bringing up running. He is already more than qualified for the unpaid internship for which he is interviewing. His writing samples are excellent, including the assignment he did for the newspaper months earlier, as a volunteer. The interview is merely to make sure that he is as responsible and capable in person as he appears on paper.

I wait a few days, maybe longer than necessary but covered by the formality of checking his references, before calling Nick to offer him the internship. He seems truly pleased to be "hired" for his first newspaper "job," and for that, I am grateful. He's a good writer, and we could really use the help.

Six months later, in June, Nick sits down in my office, having just returned home from college for the summer, ready to start his summer internship. I ask him about his term. He says it went well and that it's good to be back in Seattle, eating fresh food like avocados instead of the cafeteria glop. We exchange the bare minimum of pleasantries. Nick is as understated and affectless as before. Is he so introverted that this type of interaction is painful for him? Or is he merely reserved?

A moment passes. I pause, trying to be patient with Nick's silence, rather than chat it away. Finally, he leans forward.

"So, 3:46 in the Boston Marathon," he says, softly, almost reverently.

A surprised smile forms on my face. He has been waiting to say this. It is at once awkward and endearing and maybe a little weird that Nick has not only looked up my time but, months after the fact, he is bringing it up to discuss with me. People say that after you run many marathons, others no longer care how long it took you to finish. But some people care—other runners, serious ones, do.

Yes, I mutter. It was a warm day. I'm suddenly and inexplicably self-conscious that I hadn't run faster. Nick seems too sincere to be humoring or flattering me but something inside me won't take the chance. My instinct is to default to "all business" mode, and that's just what I do.

School-marmishly, I tell Nick that it was good experience and he should run Boston someday, when he can afford the junk miles. I guess in saying this I am attempting to acknowledge my understanding that what we do is different. His running is talent; mine is purely a midlife hobby.

There is another reason I brush off talk of the Boston Marathon. It's only Day One, yet this young man of few words has somehow managed to choose the very words that could reveal the most about me. Like a good journalist, Nick has gone to the heart of my story. But he'll be long done with his summer internship before I have the words to tell him what the Boston Marathon means to me.

CHAPTER TWENTY-EIGHT
One Boston

As Daniel and I said our vows, Dad sat front and center, arms crossed over his chest, eyes closed. Matt and Melissa had gotten him dressed and taken him to the wedding venue. I was shocked, relieved, and extremely grateful for their efforts when I saw him, slumped in brand-new khaki pants and a stiff, wrinkle-free, button-down shirt. Dad might've been nodding off, but I didn't mind. The father of the bride was here, and he wasn't even snoring.

In hindsight, it was a high point for him—for both of us, really. About two years later, I got one of those heart-stopping phone calls the children of every errant, fragile parent come to dread. Dad was in the intensive care unit at a nearby hospital. He had fallen in the tavern and lain there for hours—maybe a full day—before someone came in and found him. His wife finally called to tell me. She didn't call earlier, she said, because she thought I'd be mad.

I wasn't mad; I was livid.

At the hospital, Dad's doctor said his blood work was "consistent with someone who gets all of their calories from alcohol." So now I had what I never wanted: scientific proof of my own long-held hypothesis.

I pleaded with the convalescent center he later entered to keep him as long as Medicare would allow. I needed time to find a place for him go. After all, I reasoned, a boarded-up tavern was hardly an appropriate home for a senior citizen with a walker.

But on the day Dad was scheduled to be discharged, his wife appeared, acting as it had all been a little misunderstanding. He was going home with her; everything was settled.

"You can go now," Dad told me, sitting like a prince in his borrowed wheelchair. "I'm done with you."

I kept my distance after that. It was his life and his decisions to make. But was he done with me? Ha. Hardly.

Less than two years later, Dad called and told me his wife had moved out, and he had no idea where she went. He'd made a foolish bet and lost. I was sad to hear it and worried for him. As dysfunctional as my dad's marriage had been, it was at least a backstop for his downward momentum. With his wife gone and my brother and sister living far out of state, he had no one. No one but me.

If there was an "upside" to this, it was that the coast was finally clear. I could go visit him at his house, instead of the tavern, which had always been his true home, anyway. But I was still hurt and angry that he'd so coldly dismissed me. And now he'd be much worse off as a result.

So I didn't go see him right away. Instead, I pulled on a running shirt and wore my ambivalence on its sleeve. For fourteen miles, I turned things over in my head.

But when he didn't answer his phone for a few days straight, I told my sister Melissa and my friend Erica. Both, independent of each other, urged me to at least go check on him.

That night, I drove across town to his house, a modest little rambler less than a mile from his tavern. It was already dark and starting to rain. I pounded on the front door, then the side door. I pounded so hard my hand throbbed. He didn't answer. I called his number again, but I couldn't hear his phone ring inside.

My mind raced. It was frightening to imagine the shape he might be in when he answered the door, but even more terrifying was the thought that he might not answer at all.

I heard some rumbling coming from the basement. Then I remembered: My dad and his wife had finished it so they could rent out the upstairs. No one ever did move in, but they'd continued to live where the garage used to be, which made no sense to me.

The back porch light flicked on. I walked to the side yard and saw a flesh-colored globe; my dad's bald head peeking out of the slider. Dad was fine, he said, he'd only been sleeping. What time was it?

It was 6:48 p.m.

Things did not seem brighter when I returned in the light of day. The curtains were closed, but in the dim light, I could tell the place was a mess, like a scene from the reality show *Hoarders*. Unopened mail was littered about, PAST DUE marked on yellow and red envelopes, mingling with garbage. It looked like he'd hadn't opened anything in months, much less done any cleaning.

And that was just the living room. I dreaded the thought of entering the kitchen or bathroom.

I got back into my car and drove to the nearest store, where I bought cleaning supplies and rubber gloves, plus a box of plastic garbage bags. Back in his house, I shoved as much clutter and debris as I could into the bags and cleared off whatever surfaces I could. From the stench, disgust, and my own remorse, it was all I could do not to throw up. I made a mental note to come back with one of those face masks construction workers use and a big can of disinfectant.

Exactly how much does a person owe their parent? Every generation must solve this equation for themselves, I supposed. But it shocked me that it was now my turn, already.

Even to begin, I had to strike the word "parent," a loaded, sentimental word that never really described my relationship with Dad. This changed my perspective, allowing me to zoom way, way out, and see him not as someone who had so often disappointed me in my life but as a man who perhaps had had so much disappointment in his own.

Forget history, ancestry, our shared DNA (*Please*). None of that actually mattered. Dad was just a human being in need of help. And I was a human being who could provide it.

Since the most basic human need is food, I began showing up each week to take him to get groceries. It was disturbing to think about what his doctor said about his diet. Simple carbs certainly weren't helping his brain function. Into the cart I tossed a stack of microwaveable meals that included protein and vegetables.

Dad couldn't walk very well, due to his hip, so I suggested he use one of the mobility scooters parked inside the store's front door. Big mistake. Careening through the aisles like a NASCAR driver, he hit other shoppers so often and unapologetically that I came to suspect his crashes were deliberate.

An argument ensued the first time Dad put a bottle of whiskey in the cart. I remembered that a statewide voter initiative was the reason it was now legal for hard alcohol to be sold at grocery stores.

Had I voted for it? I had. Dammit.

At first, I stood my ground. But I wasn't his parent or guardian, and I knew that if I was going to successfully coax him out of his house and into coming with me each week, he had to be able to exert some form of control. The public health model called harm reduction would be my approach. Besides, he was paying for it. His money, his decisions, his life.

At least, I could put it all on the record, raise every available red flag. I called the state agency Adult Protective Services, spitting out all the social-service jargon I could think of: self-neglect; vulnerable adult. Everyone was sympathetic, but no one would intervene because as it turns out, it's completely legal to live in squalor, as long as it's voluntary and you hurt no one but yourself.

Six months later, in April 2013, Dad had a series of small strokes. He was taken out of his home in an ambulance about a week before I was to travel to Boston for the Marathon.

This seemed like an especially cruel blow. Though relatively minor, the strokes hit him when he was already down. He'd been paying dearly for past choices. Hadn't he suffered enough?

In the back of my mind, though, I also knew something good would come of it. In the hospital, he would get the medical care and support he needed. And he'd be there for a while, time enough for me to ensure that neither of us would ever return to that filthy house.

I wore my blue-and-yellow Boston Marathon jacket to visit my dad in the nursing home after I got back from the 2013 Boston Marathon. Despite all that happened at the race, Dad didn't ask me about it, but I didn't expect him to. He had problems of his own.

But as I was leaving, I ran into the social worker for his floor. She noticed my jacket and asked about the race and if I planned to go back.

"I don't know," I said, maybe a little too sharply.

She nodded. "Of course," she gently replied.

In the months after the race, I heard lots of people say that, given the tragedy, a marathon, with its focus on hours, minutes, and seconds, is meaningless. For a while, I started to believe them.

I finished the 2013 race fast enough to be safe, all that mattered at the time. Only later did I remember I'd done something that seemed impossible just a few years ago: I qualified for the Boston Marathon at the Boston Marathon, running 3:41:26, my second-fastest marathon ever.

When I returned to Boston after the bombing, what awaited me was yet another reminder of mortality: my dad's decline. After spending an hour or so with him at the nursing home, I often wanted to bolt from the room, get outdoors, and run as fast and as long as I could, while I still could.

More than once I pretty much did just that, having stashed my running clothes in my car because I knew that I'd emerge desperate to feel the wind in my face and long, hard breaths in my chest. I knew running wasn't everything, but it could be many things. Most of all, running was living.

My performance at Boston meant that if I wanted to, I'd be able to sign up on the second wave of the new, rolling admissions process, virtually guaranteeing my entry.

One thing that I had learned from running marathons is that no matter how good or bad you feel, at some point that will change. And it holds true: my mind changed. Or maybe it's a change of heart. I sign up. I'll officially be going back to Boston.

***

As I PICK up my 2014 race packet, the race volunteer thanks me "for coming back." No, I want to say, thank *you*.

The BAA increased the size of the 2014 field to 36,000 participants to accommodate increased interest in the race. Even at the Expo, I can see the difference in size; it's far more crowded.

I brace myself for a plethora of Boston Strong merchandise, but there isn't as much as I'd expected, and what exists is subtle. New Balance is selling a t-shirt with BOSTON as a tortuous acronym: "Because Our HearTS kept ON running."

It takes forever to wind my way around all the people crowded in the aisles of vendors. By the time I get to the Brooks booth, it's too late to see who I came for: I just missed Desiree Linden. Of all the elite women, she's the one I most want to meet. I admired her gritty performance in 2011, which I watched online afterward, from my office at work. She'd come to the race a dark horse, and though she lost to Sharon Cherop by a mere two seconds, she'd proven herself a true contender.

I had recently replayed the end of the race on my computer at work. Her performance was so thrilling to me—even though I knew the outcome—that afterward I burst into the office where my boss, Alan, was working, to tell him all about it as he sat there, looking amused.

As I exit the Expo with Dan, I see that outside the Copley T stop, a long line stretches down the block in front of is Old South Church, an imposing Gothic-style stone church known as the Church of the Finish Line.

"What could they be giving away," I slyly wonder to Daniel. "Free books?"

As we get closer, I see runners are receiving blue-and-yellow knitted scarves. I get in line for one. Behind me is a man who needs a scarf much more than me. The exposed skin of his pumped-up body is gleaming with oil and covered in tattoos. All he is wearing is a Speedo, shoes, and knee-high compression socks.

Good thing they're giving scarves away outside of the church.

A man hands me a scarf from a tangle of blue and gold in his hand.

"This scarf is interwoven with love and courage," says a yellow tag pinned to it. It's from the Marathon Scarf Project, a grassroots knitting project created by members of the Old South Church to welcome runners to Boston. The woman who knitted it signed her name: Lucy, from Weymouth, Mass.

I wrap the scarf around my neck.

Thank you, Lucy. It's perfect; better than anything I could buy at the Expo.

We don't go back to the Expo. There's no need; the scarf is all the Boston Strong I could want. Besides, the day before the marathon is time to stay off the legs. All day Sunday, my tummy churns with nerves, but when I wake up early Monday morning, the nerves have turned to excitement. It's time. I'm ready. Let's do this.

Dan walks me to the Public Garden and waits with me until it's my turn to board the bus to Hopkinton. I wish he could ride all the way with me, then laugh at myself for such a ridiculous desire. *Don't be such a baby, Amy. You've done this twice already.*

I file in and take my seat near the window in front. A young woman from Pennsylvania named Patty sits down next to me and asks if I've run this race before.

Well, Patty, glad you asked...

Now I get to play the part of a Boston Marathon veteran, here for a three-peat. But Patty's story is more moving that mine. Patty got an entry to the race through a friend, also named Amy, who had been injured by shrapnel from the explosions at the finish line.

Amy had intended for that race to be her last marathon, Patty explains, but when the BAA invited her back, she'd decided to do one more. The doctor who removed the shrapnel from her leg is also a runner, and they are running the race together today. First-time marathoner Patty is on her own.

"Well, you picked a great marathon to do, and a great year to do it," I say.

Patty continues, saying that she's nervous. Her training hadn't been what she'd hoped. There was lots of snow over the winter, and her long run topped out at seventeen miles.

"Don't worry," I say. "Once you get that far, the support from the crowd will take you the rest of the way. You'll see. It's going to be amazing."

Patty seems relieved. She keeps checking a weather app on the phone. I look away as soon as I see the big yellow sun icon. If it's going to be hot, I don't want to know.

Our bus has been sitting on Tremont Street for a long time. Finally, we start to roll forward. People on the sidewalks clap and cheer as the bus rumbles toward the freeway.

At the Athlete's Village, I get in line for the Porta Potty immediately. With thousands more runners this year, I'm in for a long wait.

"Quite intellectual reading for the moments before the Boston Marathon," says a British-accented voice from behind me.

The man in line behind me is gesturing to the copy of *The New Yorker* that, on Dan's advice, I stuffed into my clear plastic bag of pre-race items. Dan said I should have something non-running to read to calm my nerves and occupy my time.

"I guess it is," I say with a laugh. "It's a brand-new issue, and I'm going to have to throw it away when I start, but you know how it goes. There's plenty more where that comes from."

"Oh, no, you can't waste it," he replies.

Is he kidding? It's not like I'm going to run a marathon with a magazine in my hand. What am I going to do? Take a break and read "Talk of the Town" in Wellesley?

He urges me to drop the magazine off at the information table for someone else to read while they wait their turn to start the race.

I can't tell if this is dry British wit or a sincere suggestion, but I'm glad the magazine has given us something other than running to talk about. My nerves are frayed as it is.

The man introduces himself, informing me that he is an academic from the South of England, running his first Boston, and by the sound of it, also an avid reader of intellectual periodicals. He weighs the merits of the UK edition of *The Economist* versus the international one we read in the United States, and praises the *New York Review of Books*, one of his favorites.

We inch forward in line. I glance at my watch. It's already 10:25 a.m., the time I'm supposed to be headed to my corral. I haven't gotten anything more to eat or drink, and now I won't have time.

I pop a tablet of cola-flavored electrolyte into my water bottle and slug it down. Finally coming up for air, I wish the British man good luck on his race and proceed to weave my way to the corral. I probably didn't need to pee, anyway, it was just nerves. Not that I've felt nervous up to this point. The British runner and his high-minded monologue have been a pleasant distraction.

On the long walk down a picket-fence-lined street to the start, there are plastic bags or runners to deposit surplus layers of clothing.

"Goodbye, jacket I've had forever," one woman cries mock-mournfully as she peels off a windbreaker. I unzip my old H&M hoodie and toss it into a bag, along with my old black pants and even my tattered gloves. My hands are nearly always cold at the start of the race, but it's plenty warm enough to start with bare hands now.

Some guys hold a sign offering "Cigarettes, donuts, and beer." They're drinking Bud Light from cans and offering some to runners.

"If I was in my twenties, I'd do it," a man in front of me boastfully declares.

I'm so thirsty, all I want is a bottle of Gatorade. Half-empty bottles of water sit abandoned at the side of the road. I consider picking up one of them to drink.

How gross would that be? How risky? It's no good to go to start a marathon already this thirsty.

The traditional "store" where everything is free that someone sets up each year on the way to the corral is in the same spot as before. Runners are using Sharpies to write "Boston Strong" on their arms, and there's Vaseline and sunscreen but no water, nor the candy I remember. Perhaps this year, with so many more runners, the store's operator concentrated on the essentials.

I spot a bottle of water on the table.

"Can I take that?" I ask a man behind the table.

"Go ahead, I don't know whose it is."

It's unopened, so it's mine. I swig from it as I walk. I hope this liquid won't make me need to pee again. Supposedly, there are Porta Potties right near the corrals, but it's so crowded I can't see them.

I've run fourteen marathons and never had to pee during any of them. Probably I'll just sweat it out.

I follow the arrows to my corral and a volunteer checks my bib and clicks a counter as I enter. I look around at the other runners. Many of them have "Boston Strong" on their shirts.

A woman standing in front of me has printed out color copies of photos of some of the victims of the bombings and its aftermath; Krystle, Martin, Lingzi, and Sean stare back at me from underneath plastic sleeves pinned to her back.

Their faces are more than familiar. I've thought of them nearly every day for the past year. They were at the finish line to cheer on the runners. Their presence, and the presence of thousands like them, is what makes the Boston Marathon so special.

Krystle Campbell is the freckled twenty-nine-year-old from Medford with the big smile who had given up her place at the barrier so that someone else could watch their loved one cross the finish line.

Martin Richard is the eight-year-old boy whose drawing urging,

"No more hurting people. Peace," has become an iconic image, and whose parents, Bill and Denise, created the MR8 Foundation to advance compassion and kindness by providing youth with opportunities to learn, grow, and lead.

Lingzi Lü is the ambitious twenty-three-year-old from China who had been working toward a master's degree in statistics at Boston University.

Sean Collier, looking heroic in his uniform, is the twenty-six-year-old MIT police officer who was killed in the shoot-out in Watertown the Thursday after the bombing.

I remember being gripped by online news updates of the incident, horrified at the violence as it played out, virtually in real-time, online.

Sadness wells up inside of me. Anger, too, as well as fear. This is not the state of mind I wish to be in as I start the race, or at any time during the next 26.2 miles.

I feel like I might cry. But it's nearly impossible to run well while crying. I need to be able to breathe.

I want to be happy. I intend to run this race with gratitude and resilience. I've heard several people say that the Pharrell song "Happy" is their theme for the marathon. Maybe it ought to be mine as well.

If you listen to the song, it's a manic tune, bopping along gaily like a helium-filled balloon that at any moment might run out of gas. *Because I'm happy . . .* goes the chorus, over and over. This relentless insistence reminds me of Boston Strong. If we say it enough, maybe it will turn out be true.

I shuffle over a few steps. The back of the person I now stand behind has nothing written on it. His shirt is a blank slate.

Over the PA system, another song is playing. It's live; a singer-songwriter is on a nearby platform, strumming her guitar. I can barely hear her above the din of hundreds of runners talking excitedly in the corrals, but I recognize the folky song; I saw a video of it online. It's a Boston Strong-type ballad, sober and poignant. Not what I need at all.

In my head, I turn up Pharrell.

Clap along if you feel like happiness is the truth.

The crowds are already deep, even here at the start in Hopkinton. People and signs are everywhere. Some are gathered in groups, in identical t-shirts.

Kids seeking high fives line either side of the road. A big, bearded man standing atop a rock holds up a piece of cardboard shaped into the number one. "We run as one today," it says.

I smile and hold up my index finger, and he meets my gaze and says: "One Boston, that's right. You're all running as one today."

Certainly, it is a race at the front, but here in the great, wide middle of the pack, we are a unified mass of emotion, rolling together down Route 128, intent to "take back the finish line," as several signs urge.

There are references to 2013 everywhere.

"Say goodbye to heartbreak," one sign instructs, in careful Magic Marker.

"Unstoppable Boston," says another, above a silhouette of the city's skyline.

From the window of an old, white clapboard house hangs a white sheet spray-painted in black.

"This is our effing city," it says.

"Your heart didn't break," another sign says. "Don't just run strong, run Boston Strong," and "B Strong," say signs on cardboard.

On scaffolding, someone has erected a scale model of the Prudential Center. It looks like papier-mâché.

The narrow highway seems especially crowded. Many people are wearing yellow and blue. I'm rolling along in Newton when I hear a rumble in the pack around me.

"MEB WON!" someone shouts.

Wait, what? Is it true? They aren't talking about the Red Sox game, are they?

I'm a huge fan of Meb, but this seems apocryphal, almost too good to be true.

As I move along, I spot meaningful landmarks. I see the firehouse where in 2011 Ryan Hall seemed to glide over the hills. I see the hill with the newly built apartments where I saw Dan and my Mom and Dan said, "This is the race of your life."

It was, at the time. Now this is the race of my life.

The crowd in Brookline is out of control, celebrating Meb's win by cheering on the rest of us.

It must be true, if this many people are talking about it.

I'm trying to run well and conserve my energy, but I can't resist a little celebration. I hold out my palms in a "gimme some" gesture and people respond in earnest. If someone had told me it'd be like this, I wouldn't have believed it.

Meb won; an American won. It's a different race for us now.

"Go Amy," is a constant refrain; I've got the words pinned to my shirt.

I smile, pump my fist, and the crowd goes wild: "You GOT This, Amy YEAAH, Amy!"

As I'm about to go down into the underpass near Kenmore Square, I think I hear my name. But there are so many people yelling.

Maybe not. Or maybe it's another Amy.

I take the turn on Boylston, and there it is, a surreal sight, the blue-and-gold banner of the finish line. I've made it. It's not a cliché, it's the truth; I'm Boston Strong.

After collecting my medal, posing for a photo with it, and picking up the bag of post-race food, I shuffle over to the Family Reunion Area where I see Bert and her husband Glen standing on the sidewalk.

"A-may!" Bert cheers.

They're standing in a sliver of sunlight between the shadows of the downtown buildings. I join them in a warm, bright spot. Glen, who has family near Boston, ran the Boston Marathon nearly every year before injury prompted him to switch to race-walking and, with his wife, competing in Ironman triathlons. Bert has yet to qualify, although she'd like to. Every year they come to Boston for race weekend and participate in the BAA 5K, which is held on the Saturday before Marathon Monday.

Bert says they saw me just before I ran under the underpass. The "Amy" I had heard had been them yelling for me, after all.

Dan appears, throws his arms around me, then lights up as he excitedly describes seeing Meb run right by him on his way to the finish, turning around to see how big of a lead he had.

Meb had written the names of the victims on the corners of his race bib. Thinking of them gave him extra motivation to win. He said he just kept thinking, "Boston Strong," and that he wanted to win the race for the city and for the nation.

This is so different from how I approached today's race. At the start, I was unable to look at photos of the victims. I repeated the lyrics to "Happy" in my head because I didn't want to feel so sad. Dissociative running is what they call this. It worked; I ran a 3:46, a solid race on a what for me was a warm day.

But Meb, rather than try to distract himself as I did, leaned into the sadness, found strength in it. Out of tragedy, he forged a victory. It's remarkable.

Meb's win isn't my achievement, but I feel like Enid must've felt after I qualified in Eugene: a shared excitement, communal pride. We ran as one today. Meb's victory is a win for everybody.

I want to thank him, so I do it the only way I know how to contact a celebrity—on social media. Posters featuring Meb advertising Skechers, the sponsor he secured after Nike dropped him, are on bus shelters all over Boston. On the way back to our hotel, I pose in front of one, so that it looks as if I'm running just a few steps in front of the 2014 Boston Marathon champion, and tweet my thanks to Meb. I know that it's doubtful he'll respond, but I don't care. I just want to show my gratitude.

On the morning of the 2014 marathon, Dan helped me apply a heart-shaped temporary tattoo that says "Boston" to my right shoulder. It's just a giveaway from a race sponsor, but it stayed vivid for days. When the ink and adhesive finally flake away, I have a heart-shaped tan line in its place. Boston stays on my skin a little longer. It will be on my heart forever.

CHAPTER TWENTY-NINE
Cheaters Never Win

In 1980, Rosie Ruiz crossed the Boston Marathon finish line and was declared the winner of the woman's race.

Spectators and runners alike were stunned. No one had heard of her or had remembered seeing her earlier in the race. Her running form didn't look like that of an experienced runner. She'd barely broken a sweat, nor did her body show any other evidence of having run 26.2 miles. Some have said Rosie appeared "untrained," a polite way of saying she looked too heavy to have run so fast.

Kathrine Switzer, who was covering the race for television, asked Rosie probing questions about her training. Was she doing "heavy intervals?"

Rosie didn't know what those were.

When Rosie stood alongside Bill Rodgers, the men's champion, both with laurel wreaths atop their heads, Bill did a double-take. He is known throughout the running community for having an aw-shucks way about him, but even he looked like he wasn't buying it.

Eight days later, the truth came out. Two Harvard students reported to the *Boston Globe* that they had seen Rosie emerge from the crowd and jump into the race about a half-mile from the finish line.

After an investigation, the BAA renamed Jacqueline Gareau as the winner. She had been leading the women's race at mile 19 and never saw anyone pass her. To make up for what she missed, the spritely French-Canadian was invited back to Boston where she broke the tape in a joyful reenactment on Boylston Street, wearing bell-bottom pants and a striped shirt. Finally, she got the winner's medal, and applause, and her name in the history books.

Eventually, it was discovered Rosie had also cheated her way into the race where she purportedly qualified for Boston, the New York Marathon. A photographer reported seeing her on the subway; she said she was an injured runner, making her way to the finish line for help.

Nevertheless, Rosie insisted she ran the entire way in both New York and Boston. She was the perfect villain; unrepentant, "fleshy," an outsider crashing a party for elites. Her actions, bizarre at the time, were later cast as a wacky, harmless stunt, a form of performance art. One writer even called it "the best thing to ever happen to the Boston Marathon" and the "greatest hoax in sports history."

And so Rosie got her name in the history books. "Pulling a Rosie Ruiz" is now a metaphor for deliberately short-cutting a marathon course.

Whenever there is something coveted at stake, from a Presidential Fitness patch to an Olympic medal, there are those who will try to get it by cutting corners, bending or even breaking the rules. At Boston, people have cheated not just to win, but even to experience the thrill of participating in the race.

Chelsa Crowley is one of these people. A week after the 2014 Boston Marathon, someone sends me a link to a story about her.

Looking back, I should not have opened it, but I did.

Chelsa ran the 2014 Boston Marathon with a counterfeit bib, so that she appeared to be a registered runner. She crossed the finish line and accepted a finisher's medal from a volunteer. She was outed when MarathonFoto, the company that sells race pictures, sent photos of her in her fake bib number to the woman who was registered for the race under the same number.

Chelsa ran the race with her husband Dennis Crowley, who was one of the thousands offered a bib by the BAA because he had not been allowed to finish in 2013. Dennis Crowley is the founder of Foursquare, a social networking app I didn't realize still existed but has nonetheless made him rich. In 2013, Fast Company estimated his net worth as thirty million dollars.

Revelations of their transgressions set off a firestorm of criticism. In a blog post, Dennis wrote that "we" are sorry, but Chelsa, the one who wore the fake number, never uttered a digital word.

Chelsa, who is self-described as a New York fashion stylist, ran with her Twitter handle on a counterfeit bib, but after she was exposed, she didn't tweet about the race again except to note that she had tan lines from #boston going into another marathon.

So maybe Chelsa Crowley isn't sorry. Maybe she doesn't even believe she cheated but felt entitled to run the race.

The record shows otherwise: In 2013, in nearly perfect weather conditions, Chelsa, then age thirty-one, finished the Boston Marathon in 3:56, more than twenty minutes too slow for her to qualify for 2014. The time wasn't even close.

Why do people send me links to stories they know will get me incensed? More importantly, why do I open them?

Wearing a fake bib was hardly Chelsa's only option to run Boston. If the bombings were her motivation to return, as her husband suggested, Chelsa could have signed up to run with one of the many charities offering bibs to those willing to raise $5,000 to $8,000 in donations, which, given her resources, should've been a cinch. She also could have done what so many others shut out of Boston 2014 did: volunteer for the race.

The Boston Marathon is not about taking mid-race selfies for Instagram or Facebook or putting your Twitter handle on your bib. It's not about documenting your life(style) for others, it's about experiencing it, moment by precious moment. Its essence is almost antithetical to social media—it's about living in the moment completely.

It took me more than five years to qualify, and I'm grateful for all of them. It only made running Boston all the sweeter—because I deserved it. I had put in the work.

When I huddled in my car on a rainy Wednesday night and talked myself into going back out on to the muddy track to run my last two 800-meter repeats, even though I knew they'd be far slower than my training plan dictated, that was the Boston Marathon.

When I used Google maps to plot a hilly twenty-two-miler to replicate the elevation gain and loss of the Boston Marathon course, I was running Boston, already.

And when I completed my fast-finish long runs in the pouring rain, my skin rubbed raw by wet synthetic fabrics and singing songs in my head to keep my pace up, I could not have known it would be these runs, not the one from Hopkinton, that would make me worthy of accepting a finisher's medal on race day.

The more I think about it, the more I come to believe that, when she chose to wear a fake bib instead of earning a real one, Chelsa didn't cheat her way into the 2014 Boston Marathon. She cheated herself out of it.

CHAPTER THIRTY

Five Years On

I HEAD INTO the conference room and take a seat facing the window. It's a beautiful spring afternoon, and I want to be able to see outside, to the few trees and a small patch of grass visible among the downtown buildings. Everyone else does the same, until the only open chairs are the ones with their backs to the windows. You snooze, you lose.

I now work as senior writer at the American Civil Liberties Union of Washington. I've run seventeen marathons, and during this time, I've had five different jobs. I love my current one, but even so, I'd rather be out running instead of sitting through this staff meeting. The 2018 Boston Marathon is three weeks away. I've still got a few hard workouts left, and I'm antsy. I want to be out there, getting one of them done.

In meetings like these, of which there are many, I take notes to stay engaged, much the way some people focus better when they twirl their hair. Years of taking notes as a reporter have made me a prolific, compulsive note-taker. Meetings in the nonprofit world are nowhere near as fast-paced or fact-filled as press conferences, lectures, or high school debate tournaments where I honed this skill. I feel I could capture everything being said, verbatim, if I wanted to. Sometimes I try, just for the challenge.

Now it's my boss's turn to speak. He has recently announced he'll soon be retiring from his job as communications director, a position he has held for more than twenty-five years. While he is winding down his career, it seems he is more often asked to make general assessments of the state of affairs. The meeting agenda says he is going to present an overview of the Trump Administration's use of the media and its potential impact on civil liberties, a broad topic that gives him plenty of room to reflect.

He talks, I write. He is launching into an amusingly deadpan account of the many statements President Trump has made and then reneged on. Then he turns to Trump's hateful rhetoric on immigration, his relentless nonsensical tweeting, the unpredictability of presidential whims, and how media coverage of his Administration's policies might affect their eventual implementation.

Now he seems to be narrowing it to speculation of all the "Bad Things That Could Happen," which could, in turn, affect the political climate, thus making it harder for us at the ACLU to do our jobs protecting and advancing the rights of all people in America.

This is going to be a long list.

As his presentation goes on, things feel increasingly grim. *There could be a war . . .* Oh, here we go. He talks vaguely about the political impact a war could have, as if America isn't already engaged in at least two wars right now.

This reminds me: Trump hates sharks. Or at least, I read that recently. Reportedly, he even said he wished there was something that could be done about them, as if species extinction could be accomplished by Executive Order. There could be a shark attack and Trump could call for the total ban of all sharks from American waters? I sketch a shark on my legal pad, small enough that no one around me can see. Then I add a few waves for good measure.

There could be a terrorist attack . . .

The lines on my legal pad shake and blur like a computer monitor on the fritz. I get up from the table, and, in one fluid motion, swing open the door and step out of the room. I find myself speed walking to the restroom with an out-of-body feeling, as if I could look down from above and see myself moving. I should've stayed put. But leaving is not a choice I've made. My body made it for me.

I'm shocked by his boorishness. He knows I was in Boston in 2013. And he knows I'm going back in three weeks—we discussed it when he signed off on my vacation request. Even though I'd been back in 2014, it doesn't mean that I'm completely unburdened of the feelings left by 2013.

I fling open the restroom door and walk to the far stall, the large one meant for people with disabilities, lock the latch behind me, and sit down on the toilet.

I see my hands shaking. It's been five years, and yet, my breaths come fast and shallow. To slow them, I take one deep breath in and let it out gradually. As if I'm in the middle of a track workout, coming into the last lap, I space out each breath, so I don't hyperventilate.

"There could be a terrorist attack." He mentions it so casually, just talking off the top of his head. The one experience I will never be able to forget is something about me he can't be bothered to account for or even remember.

It can't happen in Boston again. Can it? A copycat?

I don't need to answer this. I need to get back to the conference room. If I return quickly, it will be as if I just had to pee and couldn't hold it any longer.

I take my seat and pick up my notepad. My boss has completed his litany of threats to democracy and is wrapping it all up with a bow. Lucky for me, I've returned just in time for the grand summation. The key takeaway, as far as I can tell, is this: No one ever knows what's going to happen. Despite the fear and uncertainty that that statement inspires within me, it's not going to stop me from going back.

CHAPTER THIRTY-ONE

No Feeling is Final

ALL NIGHT I am either too hot in the down duvet, or too cold without it. Even as I sleep, I hear the wind and the rain whipping around, or was it a dream? The squealing of the doors hinges in the hallway has me wide awake well before my alarm; people are up, rumbling around the shared kitchen, and whispering at a volume so high I wonder why they even bother. I stay in bed until the alarm sounds; I need the sleep.

I laid my whole kit out the night before, but I check the weather forecast on my phone again; still terrible. Temperatures in the thirties, a steady headwind of fifteen to twenty miles per hour, with gusts of up to forty-five miles per hour, and lots of rain, up to two inches.

The forecast has been bad for weeks, and there was talk of the marathon being canceled, something race organizers have never done. But the BAA has sent us several weather updates, reminding runners to avoid hypothermia by dressing for the conditions. If they were going to cancel the race, they probably would've done it by now.

As I head to the shared bathroom, I peer out the window in the emergency exit door at the end of the hall. Looking over the fire escape, I see rain falling into a pool of water that has collected on the roof of a nearby building. A thought pops into my mind, in an entire sentence perfectly formed: *I do not want to do this.*

It's perverse, sacrilegious, even to think this. The dread I feel is rational, but it is not actionable. Boston is more than a race, it's a pilgrimage. As long as the marathon is on, I am going to run it, and finish. It's literally what I signed up for.

Another thought occurs, one from what Enid calls the Bad Angel: "Yes, but that didn't mean you will enjoy it."

Oh, shut up Bad Angel.

Daniel and I take the T to Park Street. As we emerge from the station, rain is dumping down around us, creating rivers that pour through the streets. The grass in the park is fast becoming a muddy mess. The lines to the buses are long, but we can't even get to them because there are metal barricades all around. Additionally, the bus entry area is blocked off so that everyone must go through a security checkpoint before lining up to get on a bus. A volunteer directs us through the sloping grass to walk around to the entrance of the gate. People are walking through mud so deep it appears to be swallowing runner's shoes. Some walk up to higher ground and hold onto a fence to steady themselves in the slick conditions.

This is ridiculous, someone says, and they're right.

"Is this really the only way we can go?" I ask the volunteer. It seems precarious. I'm sorry, she says gently; it is.

A young woman turns around as she makes her way around the muddy base of a tree. It's not that bad, she cheerfully says, and motions for me to hold onto the fence so as not to wipe out. To keep my race shoes dry, I'm wearing Dan's old running shoes, which means he's wearing brand-new shoes he bought yesterday at the Expo. The bright white tread on them is already caked in brown. Reluctantly, we make it over the mud plain and to the sidewalk.

"We've got to figure something out," Dan says. At this rate, I'll be soaked before even getting on the bus.

"Let's go over there for a minute," he says, motioning emphatically, like an airport runway worker, to the Fairmont Hotel. We hurry across the street and take cover under the hotel's portico. The rain pounds loudly on the roof. Clusters of runners clad in plastic bags stand in the driveway. I pull out one of my plastic garbage bags, and Dan punches an opening in the top and helps me put it on over my head like a poncho. Punching my arms out through the plastic makes the bag split, and it falls asymmetrically over one shoulder, like Jennifer Beals's sweatshirt in *Flashdance*. I look behind a pillar and spot hotel umbrellas sitting in a stand. I grab one just as a hotel doorman walks by. He either doesn't see or is pretending not to notice. Dan grabs an umbrella for himself, and we hustle out of there.

There is a security checkpoint before entering lining up for the bus, and a guard is letting only runners with numbers in. Dan takes a couple photos of me before sending me off. My grandmother will be watching over you, he says, and we both choke up. We got a text message from his mom last night that Grandma Earsley, who has prayed for me over so many marathons, passed away. I'll be carrying her memory with me as I run.

I get in the first bus line that a volunteer would let me in, hoping not to spend too much time in the rain. Since the race organizers said only collapsible umbrellas would be allowed inside the Athlete's Village, I feared I wouldn't be able to take the large Fairmont umbrella with me. Unable to get it to collapse, I set it down on the ground.

"Are you leaving this?" someone asks. Yes, I don't think I can take it with me. Someone else says, no, I can take it, and retrieves the now-folded umbrella for me. The Hunger Games have yet to begin.

I get on the bus and head to the back, sitting in the second-to-last seat. Just like being in the green group; it's good not to be dead last. Next to me sits a young woman who is studying human factors engineering at Tufts University. Human factors engineering is just what it sounds like—engineering that accounts for our tendencies and behaviors as human animals. This whole scenario, getting people to line up, how much signage to use and where; this is like a case study in human factors, I observe.

Yes, she says, there's a whole class in how to get people to line up.

She is from Portland, Oregon, and running her second marathon as part of Tufts's marathon team, raising funds for the school and wearing a blue Nike cap embroidered with the school's name.

"I don't think I'll ever qualify myself," she says.

"Don't be so sure," I reply, hoping to give this woman a boost of confidence.

The bus ride seems to take a very long time, but I'm in no hurry to get to the Athlete's Village and be forced to wait around in the rain. When we finally pull up, I thank the driver as I leave. Runners are streaming to the entrance of the Athletes Village, but I pause. In front of me, some runners are inside the lobby of what appears to be a middle school. Are they members of a charity group who'd been offered an indoor waiting area? I walk over to check it out. I've never seen such a thing at past Boston Marathons. *A heated, indoor place to wait out of the elements? It's too good to be true.*

A security guard is stationed on a stool near the restrooms and is not letting anyone use them, but otherwise, he's condoning the runners' presence.

I find a place to sit down and chat with some of the other runners. I know that we won't be able to hear the loudspeaker announcements calling our waves to the start, so I intend to keep a close eye on the time. But before long I face a dilemma; I need to use the restroom, and the security guard isn't letting anyone in. Outside are three navy-blue Porta Potties. I was about to go and use one when I noticed they were set up at a command center for the Massachusetts state police. I ask a woman nearby if I can use them.

Another woman overhears me and points at a police officer. "He might try and stop you," she says.

"But is he a 3:37 marathoner?" I reply, only half-joking.

I don't want to give myself too much time to overanalyze. I set down my plastic bag and put a hand on the door, peering out into the rain. It isn't that far—maybe fifty yards. I just need to go.

I fling open the door and bolt for the middle Porta Potty.

"Ma'am, you can't use that, Ma'am... MA'AM. I know you can hear me!"

I don't turn to see who is doing the bellowing. I slam the door and flip the latch. My heart is pounding, more from fear than the sprinting. The adrenaline! I can't pee. There's a rumble in the box beside me, then a slam of the door. Another woman made a run for it after me—there's safety in numbers. I take my time and wait until I hear her leave. How long until it's safe to return? I imagine a cop waiting for me, arms across his burly chest. Maybe he will be angry.

I can't get arrested for disobeying an officer, can I? For unlawful use of a Porta Potty?

I wait a bit longer. Five deep breaths, same as I take each morning, eyes closed, letting my eyeliner dry. This is my final restroom opportunity before the start, as I don't want to get soaked waiting in a long line. The other woman left and I heard nothing, so I can only assume she made it back inside without incident. Drawing a deep breath of the fake air freshener air, I unlock the door and burst back into the rain, pumping my arms and driving my knees toward the middle school lobby. No yelling follows, only pattering rain. Once inside, we runners chuckle. Yet even as we're chuckling at our little rebellion, I have a sobering realization: not everyone can do this. I'm a cis-gender white woman, and so had little chance of being punished. Not everyone can be so cavalier.

A tall man clad in high-viz yellow is ordering runners to leave the building.

"You're making a mess," he says. "We can't have this."

I look around. Runners are sitting on the floor along the walls, their gear arranged around them in tidy little piles. The school's lobby is an oasis of order and cleanliness compared to the wind-and-mud strewn conditions that await us outside. But there's no use arguing. It was good while it lasted.

I gather my shoes and bags and slowly head for the exit. A young woman is fretting because she'd agreed to watch the shoes of a male runner who'd headed outdoors to relieve himself. What is she supposed to do now? If she leaves with his shoes, he'll never find her. If she puts them in the building, they might get locked up away from him. Another runner is similarly dismayed; she is waiting for her sister to join her indoors; given the weather, they'd planned to run together and keep each other's spirits up. Outside, in the chaos, how will she ever find her sister?

Meanwhile, a bus has just pulled up, disgorging more runners who now stream into the building, blocking those of us attempting to exit. They're making all of us leave, I tell one of them, but he doesn't hear me, or doesn't want to. I am glad I still have the umbrella. I open it, stepping outside.

In previous years race organizers erected a giant balloon arch over the entry to the Athletes Village, but today, all that marks the spot is a gap in the chain-link fence.

We trudge through the entrance, a sea of garbage bags and ponchos.

Twice I nearly trip on debris that is being kicked around the ground. At this rate, I will have no time to stop undercover or get any food. The distance to the starting corrals is so great, and my progress is so slow, that I must begin going there now.

But the crowd of people keeps stopping and slowing. I remember Dan telling me earlier to use "sharp elbows." I try to hold the umbrella high enough so that no one will be hit by it and beeline to the outside of the crowd, under the overhang of Hopkinton High School. Rain pours off the roof, soaking the hundreds of discarded shoes and water bottles that the oncoming runners have kicked over here, creating flotsam on a sea of mud. Stepping over them in my too-big shoes, I work my way around the edges of the crowd, thankful the umbrella that keeps me dry is also magically prompting people to yield. I need to change into my race shoes and add the ones I'm wearing to the sea in which we're swimming. But where can I do that without getting completely soaked?

Ahead, the door to a brick building opens, flashing the briefest glimpse of a vision: the inside of the gym. Is the Hopkinton High School Gym unguarded? As I approach, I see a volunteer standing outside, but she doesn't say a word.

"I just want to change my shoes," I mumble, going inside.

The Hopkinton gym is runners' nirvana. Heated and covered in shiny varnished wood the color of honey, it looks like it hasn't changed in decades. There is a nostalgic, Polaroid-photo look to the place, as if this could be any era of the Boston Marathon start line.

I'm not supposed to be here. The area is reserved for runners who are affiliated with one of the many charities that benefit from the Boston Marathon's longstanding fundraising program. These runners have raised thousands of dollars for their respective causes, while at the same time, training for a marathon.

I haven't earned this perk. All I have done for the past three months is focus on my body, and how fast I can make it go, to the benefit of no one but myself.

I plop down out of bounds on the basketball court and swap Dan's sneakers for my baby blue Nike racing shoes, locking down the skinny laces in a tight double knot. Then I grab the gel packets from my plastic bag and stuff several in my bra and one in the palm of one of the four layers of gloves on my hands.

Reluctantly, I set down the plastic bag and all its precious contents; The current week's *New Yorker*, an unopened packet of hazelnut butter, a Honey Stinger energy waffle, a complimentary banana from Tracksmith with a blue-and-yellow sticker that says Tracksmith instead of Chiquita, a fresh pack of baby wipes, a tiny tube of Vaseline. Here in the holiest of distance running sites, I make these offerings to the 2018 Marathon gods. I wish there was an altar I could place them on.

Exiting on the far side of the gym saves me crucial minutes of walking in the rain. An announcer releases the final wave of runners to go to the corrals, and they are now thundering toward me. I must stay ahead of Wave 3 or it will drown me, and I won't be able to get into my corral on time. Volunteers with plastic bags are collecting discarded clothing, but it's too early. There will be opportunities ahead, on the .7-mile walk between the exit from Athletes Village and the corrals where we line up to start.

I look for the famous "store" set up under a pop-up tent, and it's right where I remember. Rain pools on the top of the tent and drips off it. Volunteers not affiliated with the race are handing out coffee and water and have set out plastic containers of Vaseline—precisely what I am after. I applied Body Glide hours ago, while getting dressed, but in this rain, it may not be enough.

Time to lube up.

There are wooden applicator sticks scattered about so that people can serve themselves, but it's so cold that the Vaseline is nearly solid in its tub. I struggle to dig out a dollop. I try to warm it up by stirring it with a stick, then dig out a clump of the pale-yellow ointment and, hoping to be discreet, slide the stick into my shorts and spread it over my skin. I feel the warmth of my body melt the cold jelly. It's a little gross and impolite to do this in public, but, having raced in rainy weather and experienced lower-body chafing so extreme that I was afraid to even look at it, I'm willing to be indiscreet.

I grab a water bottle and have my pre-race energy gel. At the very last volunteer picking up discarded clothes, I unzip my hoodie and hand it off. I leave on my lightweight Mizuno running shell, which is eight years old and that I plan to throw away when it gets too hot. An announcer says two minutes to the start of the blue wave, my wave. I see the sign for corral four, my assigned corral, and am about to pull up my jacket to reveal my bib number for entry when I realize: I am still wearing my pants over my shorts. I hurry over to lean against the barricade and pull off my ancient Asics running pants and toss them into a bag. I enter corral four with a minute to spare and check to see that my Garmin is working. A camera on a jib swings out above our heads, and everyone smiles, cheers, and waves at whoever is watching. Now I feel good. Now I am excited.

"Okay babies," I say to everyone and no one in particular, "Warm it up and serve it hot."

We jog over the timing mats. I hit my GPS watch and the seconds start whirling. It is on.

All around me people are clad in get-ups that reveal their greatest cold weather fears. Some runners, apparently apprehensive about wet feet, run with the plastic gear-check bags lashed to their shoes. With each step, the hard plastic of the bag screeches as it scrapes against asphalt, and the blue drawstrings on the bags bounce wildly. It seems only a matter of time before someone trips on them.

Go ahead, Bigfoots. Get out of here.

Somewhere under my jacket is a yellow pace band bracelet I'd bought at the expo, marking off the splits for a 3:40 marathon. I had agonized over whether I should buy one of the bands, and if so, what pace to choose. Complicating this decision was that Boston is a hilly course, so ideal splits vary widely, but the pace bands are arranged evenly, as you would run on a course that's completely flat. I typically write splits for each mile and/or each 5K interval on my arm, but the rain made this plan impractical. A band on my wrist provides at least a guideline. I asked Dan what pace I should buy because, given the weather forecast, I wasn't sure what was realistic.

"What pace do you want to run?" he said, with characteristic (and often maddening) matter-of-factness. I hoped to be closer to 3:40 than 3:45, so I figured that was where I should aim. Shoot for the moon, and if you miss, at least you'll be among the qualifiers for Boston 2019.

The price for the yellow plastic bracelet was an unconscionable, opportunistic, ten dollars. "Do I get money back if I can't run this fast?" I asked, handing over the cash. Runners around me chuckled. Most of us would gladly fork over ten times the price if it guaranteed a certain pace.

The start is down a steep hill, so it's easy to go out too fast; nearly everyone does, including me in years past. I slow deliberately, and clusters of runners hurry by. I remember mile 1 is supposed to be no faster than 8:38. Even so, just before the mile marker, I can tell I am still going to be under pace, so I slow down drastically and hit the first mile in 8:41. I'm right where I need to be, though by putting on the brakes, I've cheated a bit to get here.

Heading into Ashland, the rain is steady, and now and again the wind whips up, rustling the plastic bags and ponchos of the runners around me.

When will I have to take off my jacket? Also: I am running a marathon in a jacket?!

I feel warm going uphill, so I unzip it but zip it back up when a biting wind rips through my two layers of clothing.

The force of the wind is pushing me back as I try to take advantage of the downhills. Miles 2 and 3 are both 8:47, a little slower than ideal, but nothing to worry about.

On the side of the road stands a man in a Santa Claus costume. Someone jokes with him that it's colder here than the North Pole.

The runners around me look excited, some perhaps a little too excited, for so early in the race. A few bob and weave to get through the loose pack. In front of me, I notice someone with a distinctive running kit; spandex shorts printed to look like denim. The "pockets" have thick stitching that reminds me of the brand True Religion. They are even embellished with a little (faux) embroidery. Déjà vu; I look at the head of the woman wearing them and recognize her super-short haircut; I've seen this runner before. During the early miles of the Light at the End of the Tunnel Marathon, where I qualified for this very race by running a new personal record of 3:37, the same trompe l'oeil jean shorts had caught my eye and left me baffled for miles. Why would anyone running a marathon want to wear clothes that suggested they were doing something entirely more casual, like attending a barbeque in the year 2000? Is there some mental benefit to dressing like a backup dancer on Pink's first world tour when you are running 26.2 miles? Enid and I always say you need to look fast to be fast, but here's someone taking what seems to be the exact opposite approach, and yet running in front of me.

With a sideways glance, I notice she is also wearing a blue headband with 2018 Boston Marathon logo in yellow. Maybe this is her first Boston Marathon. She must've qualified that day in June, in the faux jean shorts she's wearing right now.

Getting closer to her, I have the urge to say, hey we both qualified at the crazy race in Washington where you run two miles through a tunnel. And yet, how exactly does one start a conversation like that? How awkward would it be to reveal that I recognize her now because of the one day, some ten months ago, when I spent a significant amount of time staring at her ass?

A beep disrupts this train of thought: Mile 4 in 8:27.

Good. Nice. Keep it going.

Distraction, at this point, is just what I need. I can't spend too much mental energy worrying about pace. Contemplating the clothing of other runners is a much better use of my brain.

Now we are in Framingham. More people and signs line the course, many of them battered by wind and rain. A permanent sign at the side of the road is here year-round: "Proud to support all runners and victims of the 2013 Patriots Day Boston Marathon."

I straighten up, trying to run tall, with my best form and worthy of this message as we drop down and rise up a couple of inclines and declines.

Hills, in Framingham? I don't remember anyone ever talking about the Framingham hills.

Suddenly, a joyous cry from a woman's voice; "Amy, go Amy, Go AMY!!"

I look over toward the train tracks, where a petite woman huddled under a giant black golf umbrella is shouting my name. Is it my mom? No, it can't be; she is somewhere in Europe now.

"Go Amy," she repeats, as our eyes meet. Puzzled, I smile and wave, which seems to excite her; GO AMY!

Ah, I remember.

I have AMY printed in giant font on my visor, which, in a nod to the weather, I'd placed on top of a beanie. (Now it is my turn to be critiqued by the fashion police. Who would want to run the Boston Marathon looking as if their name were a headline to a breaking news story on the front page of the *New York Times*? Wouldn't a sans serif font be faster? And exactly what type of fashion statement is one making, writing their name in ALL CAPS?)

I smile to myself, both at my own hypocrisy and my obliviousness. Someone has finally obliged the request implied by the visor I've been wearing since mile 1. It took until Framingham for someone to take the hint. I feel warmed by gratitude, but I have no time to convey it.

Thank you for standing in the rain. Thank you, Framingham lady.

Framingham's train station is up ahead on the left. Townsfolk are lined up on either side of the street, behind a banner that says "Framingham Six Mile Moment."

This refers to a show the town puts on, living down its legacy as the place where, in 1907, "the race was temporarily interrupted when a train switched tracks and cut across the course, halting all but the leading six runners."

I will not be stopping in Framingham this year, but it looks like a really nice place.

"Natick with nerve" is next, and after that, mile 10. I will run mile 10 for Grandma Earsley. On Monday, Dan and I got a text message from Dan's mom: Grandma Earlsey had passed away in the middle of the night. When I spoke to Dan's sister, she suggested I run mile 10 for Marilyn, who had ten children.

"Golly," as she would say. It was an honor to accept.

The furniture store with the mirrored windows is on my right. "Check your style in the windows," a man is telling runners.

I check. My style is crap. My sopped black jacket is sticking to me in an unflattering way, and when coupled with the lavender-colored beanie and white visor I'm wearing, it makes for a crazy combination.

Lesson learned: Don't check your style on bad-weather days.

I seem to be running stride-for-stride with a man in vintage blue wind pants. He is tall, thin, and bearded, and in an age group or three ahead of me. Something about his relaxed gait makes me think he is a veteran of many a Patriots Day. He looks steady, unflappable, decisive, as if every step is landing exactly as intended and he gets a subtle satisfaction from completing each one. He isn't struggling to maintain a place in the pack, nor does he flinch when a gust of wind scours the road. I notice he is running the tangents, too, but it's like he isn't even trying.

This is the guy to run near, I think. This is a guy who knows what he is doing. His rangy frame won't block much wind for me, but I bet his rhythm is contagious.

Somewhere around a decade into my running career (if you can call it that), I started noticing runners like him. In the past I might've seen a svelte young woman with coltish long legs trot by me, ponytail swinging, and wish I had that effortlessness she seemed to project. What would it be like to be born to do this, and to look like it? Did it feel different? Can one even appreciate such a thing? A pang of envy would hit me like a side stitch, deep and shuddering, but passing in an instant. I knew these moments didn't make me jealous, only human.

But more and more, as such experiences still happened, other kinds occurred, too. In a race I'd admire the tight, economical arm carriage of a runner ahead of me, only to discover she was older—decades older— than I'd expected. I'd see the faded running shirts of veteran marathoners and be surprised that after all these years they were not just still showing up but appeared to be enjoying the events more than anyone.

It wasn't so much that a switch had flipped, more like a door had cracked open, letting in some light. Running is not only for young, thin people, but at races especially, it sometimes seems like it. Pumped-up men and tiny, ripped women in clingy shorts and neon colors may not be physically imposing, but like peacocks, when they spread their wings, they take up a lot of space.

Once, at the end of the Eugene Marathon, I spoke to a man in his eighties who came in just behind me. I asked him the secrets to running longevity. He said to do no more than two marathons a year (spring and fall), and then asked my age. I was then in my late thirties, and he told me I still had lots of time to get faster. I was happy to hear that, and he turned out to be right, but what stayed with me was the enjoyment he seemed to get, well past his fastest days.

To be like the younger runners around me just seems far-fetched. I'm too large, too ungainly, with no real talent, but increasingly, I hope to be one of the greyhounds: quiet, elegant, no effort wasted and no one to impress, running only as hard and as far as ever I please.

Next we run over Lake Cochituate, a reservoir. There is water on either side of us, and the wind off the lake cuts through my jacket. The few people gathered in this wind, cheering us on, warms me back up in the meantime.

Mile 7 is 8:54; mile 8 is 8:56.

My slowing pace is telling me something, but the question is, what? The backs of my legs are already starting to tighten. I decide not to think about pace for a bit. Wellesley is coming up. The women of Wellesley will give me a boost.

They say you can hear the Scream Tunnel from as much as a mile away. So far, all I hear is the roar of the wind. I have trudged through so many unavoidable puddles that I am no longer shocked by a plunge of cold water that soaks the thin knit uppers of my shoes. It drains out just as quickly as it came in, like the tide going back out to sea.

The Wellesley Scream Tunnel is still unmistakable to me.

I look for the funny signs, but most have fallen to the ground. The lore is that seniors at this women's college must get a kiss one of the marathon runners. It comes from a time when almost all the runners were male (and assumed to be heterosexual) and the students were assumed to be heterosexual. As such, most of them begin with "Kiss Me," as is tradition.

This year there is the inevitable: "Kiss me, I'm wet."

Bedraggled as their signs have become, the youthful exuberance is especially touching today. By now I am certain this is turning out to be one of the absolute worst weather days for spectators in the history of the race, which means for the history of this Wellesley student body and its seniors. Nevertheless, we are all out in it.

Or most of us. The numbers at Wellesley are diminished from what I remember from 2014. I don't want to kiss anyone. But the students are so emphatic that I long to somehow connect with them. If Wellesley is still going to cheer for me despite the conditions, then I'm going to cheer right back.

I hold out my hand, clad in four layers of gloves now swollen with water, and move over toward the barricades. Mustering my best varsity "Woo!" I accelerate down the right side of the road, gently slapping every hand in my way. Hands appear out of nowhere, and I high-five them with pride, like a basketball player coming off the bench to make the game-winning play. I'm smiling, but it must look like a grimace. Despite that, the cheers seem to get louder as I approach.

As soon as it is over, a few steps away, my legs burn. I just used up a lot of energy, and I'm not even halfway through the race. I have broken one of my cardinal marathon-running rules: overexuberance leads to overexertion. Maybe it does. Maybe it's worth it.

The Scream Tunnel comes near the entrance to the town, and Wellesley proper still takes up several miles. I still have quite a stretch before getting to the Newton Hills. The exhilaration has evaporated; my legs feel heavier than ever as I trudge toward the picturesque Wellesley Center.

It reminds me of my alma mater Hampshire College, which is located west of here, in the Pioneer Valley, one of five colleges that dot the pastoral landscape. Coming years ago from the big box stores and freeways of rainy, suburban Seattle into a community dotted with brick buildings and burnished autumn leaves seemed unreal. It felt like I'd been set down in a Hollywood soundstage for colleges from the 1950s.

Wellesley has the same, small-scale town center. There is an elegant stone church and boutique storefronts of red brick and white paint. Spectators surround the metal barricades of the tidy downtown, and I feel my pace quicken, and I try to tighten up my form. *Look alive*, I say to myself.

I am, but barely. In Natick, my pace slipped over the 9-minute mile barrier, and though I had dipped back under it entering Wellesley, to an 8:55 mile, my legs are getting heavy. The runner who had planned to run a 3:40, where is she? There is still a lot of race left before I get to Boston.

I need to focus.

I search the faces of the spectators lining the main street. A group of young women has gathered, hoods up on their rain jackets. One holds a small white piece of cardboard on which she's scrawled in Sharpie: "Desi won."

Desi won. WAIT . . . Desi won the Boston Marathon? It is already over, and Desiree Linden has done it?

In disbelief, I go back. Heads covered and hunched over, the women remind me of pilgrims who have traveled a great distance to bring the good news.

"Desi won?" I ask the woman, seeking to confirm, like any good journalist would, because you can't believe everything you read. She grins and nods, and I throw my arms around her, screaming "Oh my god, oh my god! Desi won! She did it! Oh my GOD!!"

I hug all the women with her, still screaming, tears welling up in my eyes.

Unbelievable: The dark horse at Boston for six years running has broken the tape, ending the drought. I know all about the odds she faced. In a stacked field of the world's best women marathoners, that Desiree Linden had become the first American woman to win at Boston since Lisa Larsen Weidenbach in 1983 is incredible. As I was dreading my own race, I had a gut feeling that the terrible conditions were perfect for a self-described gritty runner like Des, an underdog with whom I identify, but her actually winning was too much for me imagine. I didn't want to jinx it for her.

And now I'm dying to know exactly how she pulled it off. I can't wait to find out, but of course, a huge obstacle stands in my way, more than thirteen miles through the lashing wind and dumping rain. Before I can get the story of Desi's Boston Marathon, I must complete my own.

To say I am invested in Desi's race is an understatement. Of all the runners out there, even Boston-bred sweetheart Shalane, I most wanted Des to win. I've followed her career since her Boston debut. I'd began getting up early to watch the Boston Marathon years before I even had a chance of qualifying. This has made me invested in the outcomes of elites almost as much as my own.

These parallel interests could now intersect. Des's historic win should inspire me to get it together and run the last half hard.

I've got to use this; how could I not?

As I run over the halfway mat I check my time: 1:57:01. Nearly ten minutes slower than where I should be to meet my goal time. But still, under two hours, which means if I stay consistent, I could break four hours. Which isn't that bad, in these conditions.

Try to stay positive. Don't judge the race until you are done running it.

The spectators are bunched on the side of a road that curves up yet another hill. My clothes are heavy with water. I wish I could stop and wring them out. Suddenly, cold water splashes into my crotch. It's as if someone took one of the green cups of Poland Spring water being handed out at aid stations, stuck a couple of ice cubes in it, and, with remarkable aim, chucked it right between my legs. After the initial shock, I am mortified; how dare the rain touch me *there*?

Sometime later, it happens again. I wince as the water hits, then trickles down my inner thighs. It is probably only a small amount, but it's Arctic cold. I've heard of mud runs that subject participants to perilous obstacles, like placing tacks on the course. But people sign a waiver for such stuff, consent to it. Here such hazards appear without warning.

I realize that somewhere in my midsection (The bottom of my bra? My stomach?) water is collecting. I hope it is collecting in my clothing, not on an actual ledge of flesh, and though I do not wish to create a visual, it probably goes something like this: The volume of liquid eventually becomes too great for the surface it occupies, and overflows, like a colonial waterwheel, dumping into my running shorts.

I glance around, relieved no one seems to be able to tell. Of course, how could they? Drenched runners are everywhere. Rivers of rainwater careen across the road. That a diverted stream is occasionally cascading into my private parts thankfully goes unnoticed by everyone but me.

It's so cold. My mind wanders.

Run faster and you'll warm up. Shorten your stride, and the legs will turn over faster. Cadence is what you can control, when you can't think about speed.

Desi won, Desi won. Use that to fuel you. But if Desi won, it means the race is already over. No, don't say that, YOU'VE still got a race ahead of you. Just run this mile, just run the mile you're in.

A commotion interrupts this argument I'm having with myself. Some kind of yelling. I look to the side of the street and see a black umbrella bobbing above the heads of onlookers. In the spaces between people standing along course, I glimpse Dan running, holding the Fairmont umbrella aloft like Mary Poppins, shouting; "Desi won! Desi won! Amy! Amy! Desi won!"

Warmth blooms in my chest; Daniel is here! He'd told me that, given the conditions, he probably wouldn't go out on the course, but instead wait with our friends Glen and Bert, who always station themselves at the corner of Hereford and Commonwealth Avenue, near the final turn onto Boylston.

But instead, magically, Mr. Poppins has appeared.

I run to the side of the road. Onlookers move over to make space for him to meet me at the metal barrier.

"I know," I shout over the crowd's roar and the rain when he tells me again that Des won, "it's amazing!"

I lean over the barrier. Holding the umbrella high, Dan gives me quick peck on the lips. As we kiss, I can smell his skin. I can smell the rain on his soaked blue jacket. His eyes look watery and rimmed in red—as if he's been crying or needs to change his contacts. I don't want to leave him now, but I must. If I stop too long, I'll end up walking.

I retake my place in the stream of runners. I don't look back, lest the sight of his face undo me.

"Don't forget to eat!" Dan calls as after me. "Remember to eat!"

Ah, shit. Busted. I am overdue for an energy gel but have already eaten the ones in I'd tucked into each glove. All I have left are now stuffed in my sports bra, under my zipped-up jacket and long-sleeve shirt, out of reach for my inoperable hands.

Fortunately, it is not long before an aid station appears; volunteers in red jackets are handing out Clif Shots. Someone hands me a pink one, raspberry. I take it in both hands; my fingers are numb. I don't want to drop it.

I've got the Clif Shot, wet plastic slippery in my palm. But with ten digits that might as well be marked "Out of Service," despite four pairs of wet gloves, I've got no way to open it. Earlier, I opened energy gels with my molars, but that was back when I still had enough dexterity to start a tear in the plastic. I can practically hear Dan admonishing me to eat.

I am not making good decisions. Even without looking at my watch it's clear I'm slowing down. I acknowledge that this is a choice my mind is making, cowing to my body's simpering accumulation of complaints. Some fuel could help my mind fight back, give it the gumption to tell my body to stop slacking off.

Legions of red-jacketed volunteers are stationed along the course, waving energy packets at approaching runners. Above them, tall red flags identifying the color-coded flavors flap crazily in the wind. I stop in front of an unoccupied volunteer and hold up my Clif Shot.

"Can you open this for me?" I plead, but she demurs, her hands aren't working either and points to a large male volunteer a few feet away.

Exasperated, I run over to him: "Can you open this?" I say, more as an order than a request. He starts opening the Clif Shot in his hand.

"No, *this* one!" I say, thrusting my packet at him. He laughs, takes it from me, and tears it open with an effortless flick of his wrist.

"Thank you!" I say, extra cheerfully, trying to make up for barking orders at him and for my senseless insistence that he open my packet, instead of whatever greenish-yellow flavor he already had.

Who cares what flavor it is? Geez, Amy, why can't you be more polite?

In penance, I suck it down without water. It sticks in my throat, making me cough, which is funny because it tastes like cough syrup. Mr. Poppins was right; I needed to eat. Just a spoonful of sugar helps the medicine go down.

The Newton Hills must be looming, but all I can see is the road in front of me, slick with rain. Earlier in the race, on the steep downhill into Ashland, I tripped on something slippery on the ground. I managed to recover and stay upright, but it threw me off my stride.

"Oh, watch out," another runner said, sounding sincerely concerned. Ever since then, I've been aware that my Nike Vaporfly shoes, while fast, are also precarious on wet asphalt. I have to be careful in them, and the conditions are even sloppier now.

Newton makes me think of Ryan Hall, who I'd seen at the Expo just before his legendary run. When I later watched the race, I saw him flying around the hills in Newton, in his red-and-blue singlet, golden hair ruffled by the breeze and shining in the pale morning light. Bounding up the hill next to the Newton fire station, darting through shadows cast by skinny, leafless branches, Ryan made Marathon Monday look easy, a Sunday run in the park.

The Newton Hills are not easy. Everyone always talks about Heartbreak Hill, the crescendo, but the reality is that Heartbreak starts as a series of inclines that begin after you pass through the center of Newton. I thought of these hills as I trained. In anticipation, I packed my long runs with as many hills as possible.

Dan's sister, Catherine, has asked me to run mile 22 for her, as it's her favorite number. She wasn't about to pick some easy mile in the single digits. But okay, I said. I'll make it a good one. At least 22 is flat to downhill.

Catherine's request prompted me, unthinkingly, to ask Dan what part of the race he wanted me to run for him. Immediately I regretted it, because Dan is never one to make things easy. He paused only a beat before responding: "What mile is Heartbreak? I want you to run Heartbreak for me."

That my husband chose the course's most notorious point is to be expected. You always hurt the ones you love. The problem with running Heartbreak Hill with any intention is that it's unclear, even to repeat Boston Marathoners, where Heartbreak starts. There are so many hills in Newton that you can't be sure you are running Heartbreak, or a prelude to it, until you reach the top, at Boston College, and see the maroon-and-white inflatable arch that says, "The Heartbreak is over."

As soon as we begin climbing, runners on either side of me slow to a walk, rubbernecking back and forth on the course.

Don't even think about it.

My time goals may be slipping but I intend to keep running, however slowly. There is a critical difference between running and walking, though it doesn't always look like it from the outside. Conceding to walk in a marathon is something I have not done for many years now, because whenever I have, it has been a downward spiral, a road to a hole so deep I've never been able to climb back out. The road to marathon hell is paved with the good intention to begin running again.

In this view, I'm in good company. Haruki Murakami, my favorite novelist, has written about races in which he'd made and honored the same pledge. He has joked that on his tombstone there would be the inscription "At least he never walked."

This is the Boston Marathon, a runner's race if there ever was one. Maybe now I am only jogging it, but at the end of the day, I will at least be able to say the same.

But how should I accomplish this? I remember the hill running form from my drills with Chuckit years ago: shorten your stride, pump your arms to propel you up the hill, steady effort, eyes in front of you. Don't look too far up the hill, but just in front of you. I run hills all the time. I like hills. Hills are my friends.

My watch beeps with a mile marker. I try not to look at it.

Don't look, don't look, do not look.

I have always found the hardest part of marathon running is to do it without a constant internal monologue assessing how I am doing, and this is especially true when I sense I'm not doing as well as I'd like. I can tell am doing poorly now; knowing precisely how poorly probably wouldn't help.

And it doesn't.

My watch shows a ten-something pace for the mile I just completed. To have crossed a barrier that even in bad weather I never even imagined I would approach horrifies me.

But it's fine, Amy, you are running uphill. Don't look. Don't walk; just run. Naturally, you will be slower, you are running uphill. You'll make it up on the downhill. Just keep going.

I have much better mantras, so many of them, but they escape me now. My hands hurt. Digging deep inside myself is not possible, I've got no shovel. And my mind is as numb as my fingers.

So instead of digging inside, I look outside. Dissociative running, experts call it. Look at the people, their faces. As soon I make eye contact, they light up. They are happy to help; it is what they are here to do. They are enduring the same rain, buffeted by the same blasts of wind, probably for as long as I will be today. And they're not even going to get a medal at the end of it.

So many times, I've cajoled myself through the hardest parts of workouts by saying "This is the Boston Marathon, Amy."

Merely by reminding myself that training is not separate from the Boston Marathon, that they are one and the same, I transform an ordinary workout into a special occasion. There can be for me no Boston Marathon experience without the months of preparation that imbue it with importance.

I did not diminish the power of this tactic by using it needlessly. Only to psyche myself up for a final repeat, for the last tempo interval, or the last two miles of a twenty-one-mile run, when my legs ached, would I venture to say to myself, "This is the Boston Marathon, Amy. This is it, right now, not several months and eight thousand miles away but right here, right now, today."

It is remarkable how well this tactic works. Surprisingly, I often find a little more energy left in me, miraculously run one precious second faster than the goal pace that had seemed far out of reach, muster the energy to speed up at the end of a long run on which I had long since faded.

And so, here I am, Patriots Day, finally *in* the Boston Marathon, astonished to find I feel nowhere near as powerful or excited as I did on those runs alone in the Washington Park Arboretum, with no one but the chirping birds to witness my triumphant performance. How did I manage to summon my strength then? How can I channel it today?

I hear my name, as if I'm being roused from a dream. Somehow I have trash-talked myself halfway up the final Newton Hill. I figure this out because shouting at me is a young man who is, incongruously, sporting giant sunglasses and a tank top (is he really, or am I just delirious?).

"You're CRUSHING Heartbreak Amy. You're CRUSHING IT."

He is leaning over to say this to my face. He is getting up in my business to applaud me for taking care of business.

I want to laugh at his frat-boy enthusiasm, a white lie endearingly unsullied by reality. I am not crushing anything, but by confirming I'm nearing the top of Heartbreak Hill, young Mr. Tank Top has come in right on cue. Daniel knew exactly what he was doing, picking this part of the course as the part to run for him. Love hurts.

My embarrassed grin has encouraged the young man to keep cheering for me, and now others are joining in: "Amy! Woo, Amy! Yeah, Amy!" My name is everywhere. My visor is like a marquee: the Boston Marathon, starring AMY.

Students drinking beer from plastic keg cups on the side of the course without any apparent fear of hypothermia are calling it now, "Yeeeeah, Amy! You got this, Amy!"

I feel as though I am barely moving up the steep pitch. I must look on the verge of collapse, but you wouldn't know it from the accolades I'm getting. There is no way I can live up to all this adulation, but at least I've got to run strong up this final crest of the hill. I've got to pick up my feet.

The brick buildings of Boston College form the backdrop to this madness. I look up, searching for the sign.

It's up. I thought they might've not put it up this year, due to the wind, but "The Heartbreak is Over" is spelled out in inflatable letters near a blue-and-yellow course marker that reads mile 21.

The crest of Heartbreak Hill is a huge party, one of the liveliest parts of the course, but anyone who has had a difficult day at Boston knows the hardest miles are ahead.

Absorbing the chaos around me, I don't even look at my watch; I just prepare to pound the downhills. Finally!

"It's all downhill into Boston," someone shouts.

This is the point where you unhinge your legs. This is the Boston Marathon, Amy.

Ten kilometers left, just a run around Lake Union. This is where I can make up some time I've lost. Using the downhill running form I practiced over the last two months, I focus on keeping my arms low so that I don't over-stride, running comfortably.

Comfortably? Well, maybe not. My legs alternate between numbness and aching. The water-splashing thing is happening again, as if I'm wetting myself.

No one can see it, though. No one can tell.

My eyes seem cloudy, like fogged-up car windows, and I'm desperate to drive home. Things darken; we are running straight into a storm cell. It must be midday, lunchtime, maybe, but there is the ambiance of one of my winter long runs in Seattle, where even in the middle of the day it feels like the end of the world.

I feel fine.

I smile at the onlookers. Smile, run, keep smiling.

But I cannot smile at the sight now in front of me. Two police officers carry a slight man in shorts and a singlet, holding him horizontally, as if he's on an invisible stretcher. They're taking him off the course. He doesn't move. They are in high-viz yellow, and he's wearing electric purple shorts that look like part of a pro or collegiate running kit.

He's not moving! They're taking him away! But he's okay. No one is dying out here. It's fine.

Darkness is setting in. I've been running all day. It must be twilight. This feels like it is a gothic Boston Marathon. We've run from twenty-first century Boston all the way to Victorian London. Somebody fetch a match for the gas lamp.

I look at runners beside me, my fellow ragamuffins, urchins, and street people. Their bedraggled clothes are familiar. I've seen them earlier in the race.

This my pack. They haven't left my side. These are my people. I must stay with them.

Someone is standing at the side of the road, shouting something, an announcement. A bit closer, and I can tell he's saying something about a church.

This is getting maudlin; are they praying for us? No, he's saying the church is open for runners to come in and warm up. They have hot drinks, food.

Wait, what? Are they calling off the race? Are people leaving? I try to make sense of this: a warm, dry place to rest. With hot drinks and food, on the Boston Marathon course. This is not an aid station, it's purgatory.

If you leave the course, you can't come back—at least according to the official rules of the race. I remember the runner being carried off by cops and the crowded medical tent I saw a few miles ago.

Perhaps this is necessary; maybe conditions have gotten so bad that race organizers have sought help from the community. I am well-dressed for running in the elements and yet painfully cold; other runners must be freezing. But are they abandoning the race? Is this a running mutiny?

I need to put this behind me. I mustn't contemplate the possibility. The people at the church no doubt have good intentions, but we know how those can go. Stepping off the course is not an option for me, and despite how well-meaning the offer, I wonder if anyone extending it fully appreciates the temptations it creates and the consequences that could flow from them.

How many runners now inside, as warmth returns to their fingers and toes, and blood starts flowing better to their brains, will be chilled by the realization that they dropped out of Boston. They are done. It is over. DNF (Did Not Finish) will be listed online, printed next to their names in the record book for the 122nd Boston Marathon, which is mailed to every race entrant. How many will go home tormented by the thought that maybe, just maybe, they might've been able to make it?

Shuffling along, I hit what must be Cleveland circle. I step carefully over the train tracks. The white foam soles of my shoes are slick. I don't want them touching wet metal. Mounds of plastic—ponchos and garbage bags discarded by runners—blow about the course like desert tumbleweeds. A huge puddle covers the middle of the road. Most runners, me included, have no choice but to slosh right on through.

A young woman looks intently at me: "Finish the job."

She is saying this to everybody, but as she meets my gaze, it's as if she's pressing her message deep into my consciousness. This I appreciate.

This is useful. Telling me I am crushing it is kind yet laughable. Instead, she projects an authority that makes believe she, too, has struggled on a marathon course, maybe this one. Respectfully, she is asking only that I get this done.

"Finish the job," she repeats.

It's the minimum, and right now, that's everything.

At this point, the course is running alongside the MBTA train tracks. Kenmore Square is somewhere up ahead. I can't wait to get there. I can't wait to see the Buckminster Hotel, where I stayed when I first came to Boston before heading off to college, and several times since.

The Buckminster is lucky for me, waiting up ahead. I need to get there. How far is it? Just get to the next mile.

I look for the Citgo sign, which is two miles away from the finish. When you run by it, you are one mile away, but the rain is making it hard to see more than a few feet in front of me. I can hear plenty, though. People are more vocal than they have been since Hopkinton.

So much yelling; it's an aural assault. The collective din overwhelms me, makes me feel weepy and weak. I listen for individual voices, trying to sort them out. This helps. It's not an angry mob; these are my fans, come to cheer me on in my rock-star moment.

Where are we? All I can see are some brick buildings. That's a lot of help. Brick buildings are everywhere in Boston. Oh, and a hospital, but same thing. Hospitals and universities, you could be almost anywhere on the whole damn course.

My right foot hurts. I have a toenail that always bruises black in races, so I'm wearing a silicone cap to protect it. Now I feel the toe cap touching the top of my shoe. It is a weird sensation, my toe is swollen and tender from running downhill, slamming against my shoe, and the cap feels like it's coming off. But it's not because I wear it in training and it feels the same way at the end of a long run.

This is nothing new, and it's fine. Just keep running. Finish the job.

Up another hill, an overpass, and immediately, people drop to a walk, including the runner right in front of me. Normally this aggravates me, but I no longer have the energy to be aggravated. I just run (okay, jog) around him. My serpentine, time-wasting path through the people who are walking makes it seem that in comparison to them, I'm absolutely conquering this rise. I know it's only an illusion, but it's one I can put to good use.

I am finishing the job.

This is the last hill, other than the underpass—Mt. Hereford, as Kara Goucher once called it. Just get on up, and I can glide right down. Pound the downhills, pound the downhills, damn the torpedoes and my aching legs.

One more mile, just run this one. Which mile is this? No idea. Can't see the mile markers. Did the wind blow them down? Doesn't matter. I'll know the turn when I get to take it, I'll know I'm about to take the sweetest right turn in the world; right on Hereford, left on Boylston. It's up there somewhere. Just keep going.

Finish the job.

The rain is pounding down and yet the hundreds, no, thousands of people standing to greet us are also getting hammered, and they're not even moving to keep warm.

Oh man, the crowds now. Either side of the road.

Rain is dumping so hard that a woman running beside me cackles at the absurdity, and I chuckle, too. The marathon gods are playing us all for fools. Water splashes back up from the pavement. I laugh a little, too, but my gut hurts. No laughing, no crying, just keep running.

And smile: Eureka, the Citgo sign! I'm going to run right under it. We are in Kenmore Square, must've passed the Buckminster and Fenway and Kenway back there, but I missed all of them. A race photographer is crouched at the side of the road, so in their race photos, runners will have the Citgo sign right behind them. I run over to him, pull up my jacket to reveal my race bib and give him best smile-grimace.

Finish the job.

Down under the underpass; not a sound from the crowd. It's not dry so the slapping of feet against wet pavement echoes, and I can hear all of us breathing. Six seconds of air going in and out of my lungs and we are back out into what passes for daylight, into the relentless wind. I lean into the hill, pull my arms high and tight to my body to propel myself up this final incline.

One kilometer to go, way less than a mile, so it's time to move to the right side of the road. AAAAAAMMMMMYYYYY! Daniel and Glen and Bert are yelling at me from the side of the road. I see them as if in stop-motion, each of their faces held up to the rain. I yell back at them and keep going to the corner of Hereford.

Right on Hereford, this is it. This. Is. The Boston Marathon, Amy!

After miles of villages, I have arrived in the city. The buildings tower over me, like I'm an ant in a canyon.

I want to run the tangents, but there are too many people on my left. I can't get over in traffic, so I run straight down the short block called Exeter. The Hynes Convention Center looks like a cartoon wall ahead; right at it we run, then turn 90 degrees before slamming into it.

Up ahead, the finish line is draped in yellow and blue, but the rain makes it look tiny and remote, an island on the horizon. It's an illusion; I know all of this will be over in the blink of an eye.

Up on my toes, pumping my arms, I am no longer a marathon runner, I'm a track athlete now, surging into the final stretch.

This is the Boston Marathon, Amy.

My turn goes wide, I pump my arms and churn my legs faster than I have for too many miles. Festooned in blue and yellow, Boylston is as loud as a football stadium. The runners you see in books and magazines and on TV, powering down a final straightaway to the deafening adulation of adoring fans, that's me, that's everybody. People on the streets are probably calling my name, but all I hear is a muddle of sounds echoing off the buildings.

The finish line still looks far, but I know it's practically behind me. My legs must be doing their job on autopilot, I can't feel anything in my body.

On the ground, I see three blue stripes. They trace the shortest route to the finish. There are two mats at the finish, and most people slow down when they hit the first so that by the second they are coming to a full stop. But I hit the first mat with such momentum that I'm in mid-stride going over the second. When I run, the man in front of me stops to walk, I slam on the brakes to avoid crashing into him.

Finally, I made it. Amid hundreds of other sopped, relieved runners, I've finished my fourth Boston Marathon. Volunteers hand out water bottles, having thoughtfully loosened the caps. Here we are, in the Promised Land. I take a long swig.

Finally; it's over. I'm beaming at the volunteers, other runners.

But where are the medals?

Never have I wanted a finisher's medal so badly. I haven't even kept all the race medals I've gotten over the years. But I need this one.

Here is a volunteer, presenting a medal to me. I beam as she loops the medal around my neck and congratulates me.

I thank her and spot a photographer waiting. The fans, the paparazzi of Boston; they just won't leave me alone. I stride toward the camera like it's the red carpet at the Oscars. In one hand, I grip my bottle of Poland Spring, the champagne of the finish line. With the other, I pull up my drenched black running jacket (I'm wearing Mizuno, my favorite designer) to show him my bib and give my best Hollywood smile, like, "I didn't win the Boston Marathon, but it's an honor just be nominated."

A few steps forward and someone drapes a foil blanket around me and affixes it in the front, like a parent putting a superhero cape on a child. I swaddle myself in the heat sheet, trying to reverse the effects of stopping so soon. Lightheaded, I need to keep walking.

At the gear-check tent, I recite my race number like a poem I've known since childhood. The gear-check bag can be worn like a backpack, but I just clutch it under my foil poncho and toddle toward the family reunion area, wherever that might be. "Where's the family reunion area?" I keep asking volunteers, and they give complex, multi-step directions.

Why so complicated? Is it still even in Boston?

Finishers are being wheeled around in wheelchairs.

Looks nice, getting a ride like that.

I get to the intersection where the volunteer told me to go.

"Where's the family reunion area?" I plead with a red-jacketed man. "Okay, just go down to the blah blah blah…"

I'm cold; the steps I take are tiny. A bitter wind blows up my heat sheet, making a mockery of its name. A woman shuffles past; her lips are blue; her face is grey. She looks terrible, like the victim of a catastrophe. But the volunteers can see her too, and they do nothing. So maybe she's already gotten the help she needs?

Race volunteers, or maybe officials, or maybe medical people, are sitting on tall chairs that remind me of lifeguard chairs. From their perch, they make announcements into battery-powered megaphones. Probably they're also keeping an eye out for people who faint in the streets.

"Congratulations, Amy," says a voice from above.

It's a woman in one of the chairs, interrupting her race announcements to give me a shout-out. My personalized visor is still working its magic, well past the finish line.

Maybe I should take it off now. Or maybe I should wear it every day for the rest of my life. I'll be at my desk at work, struggling with a tricky bit of writing, and a colleague will walk by and say, "You got this, Amy." I'll pop on the visor and walk past the front desk of the assisted living facility where my dad lives, and the woman at the sign-in sheet will say, "It's all you, Amy." I could get used that.

A giant yellow-and-blue sign appears: Family Reunion Area. Dan and I thought we were being smart by choosing to meet at A for Amy instead of R for Roe. But somehow, I walked smack-dab into the middle of the alphabet.

Which way is A? How do the letters go?

I see Dan waiting.

"We've got to get you warmed up," he says as we embrace under the trusty Fairmont umbrella. I'd heard an announcement about a warming station, but I can't imagine what such a thing might look like, much less find it. I tell him about it, and he trots off, leaving me shivering and alone.

The warming station is a charter coach parked on the street right in front of us. We board the bus, take seats near the back, and I never want to leave.

The bus is half-full, brand-new and aggressively heated, its upholstered seats soft and plush. We started the day on a school bus, but this is a bus for another life stage: retirement. I'd like to recline the seat and take a nap. I'm ready to enjoy my Golden Years.

Dan is having none of it. "Change out of your clothes," he barks, all tough love.

I contort my tender limbs to strip off my wet gear and put on the clothes from my gear-check bag. In the cramped space between seats, the process is painstaking. Trying to stay covered by the heat sheet for modesty's sake, I take my time. Finally, I'm in no hurry.

"You need to eat."

I'd tried to eat a Clif Bar after finishing, but it was frozen so hard I feared I'd break a tooth. Like a baby, I want to refuse all food.

In my bag are King's Hawaiian sweet rolls, the same sustenance I chose in 2013. Soft enough to go down easy, they are biscuits for teething. I eat all four from the package, hoping this will satisfy Daniel. If this bus had some hot coffee, it would be nirvana. Just put it in my bottle.

A man who has changed from his running gear is standing in the aisle talking about how epic the race was, and how terrible the conditions were, loudly repeating, "You have no idea."

Excuse me, sir, I have much more than an idea—I know precisely what it was like.

"No, you have NO IDEA," he bellows again, as if answering my thoughts. He is standing in the aisle talking on his phone, but it's as everyone on the bus is his audience.

I don't need to be reminded of what we just went through. The gratitude I feel to be inside a heated charter bus, wearing warm, dry clothes, Daniel at my side lovingly ordering me to eat, this is all I wish to inhabit. But the man won't stop broadcasting his recollections; the rain and wind, the specific misery he alone experienced. His voice is so loud, and I feel so sensitive. You have no idea.

Present hedonist that I am, I intend to luxuriate in the moment, looking neither back on the race, nor beyond it. The bus is a buffer from the outside world, a liminal space. The race clock has stopped, yet the gravity of the Boston Marathon keeps me in her orbit. If only I could stay here forever.

As soon as we exit the finish area, and I shower off the sweat of my effort, put on clean clothes and my race jacket and medal, I will reenter the normal world, Planet Earth. Then my race experience will be rationalized. I will have no choice but to look back on it, evaluate the data, and make a case for and/or against my performance.

I completed the 2018 Boston Marathon in 4 hours, 13 minutes, and 22 seconds, in 18,258th place. It is the slowest marathon I have run in nearly a decade, more than thirty minutes slower than my goal of 3:40.

That I started the race on goal pace was my first, most egregious mistake. But in the hours leading up to the start of my wave, I'd done such a good job avoiding the elements that I arrived at my corral all but unscathed. Had I stood for an hour or two, in a field of mud, under a tent battered by thirty-mile-per-hour winds, I might've come to the realization that we had been given D-minus weather conditions in which to run, and it was woefully unrealistic for me to start out at my A-plus pace.

But that wasn't my only stumble. During the middle miles, when my pace began to slip, I accepted this slippage, rather than digging in to counter it. The wind and rain were unrelenting, but my own emotions buffeted me most. I whipsawed between indignation at the weather, shock and confusion at what was happening to my own body and the bodies around me, and a fragile resolve to get back on track. With goal times out of reach, I struggled to stay engaged with the race and my reasons for running it.

As the weather worsened, so did my outlook. By the time I got to the point on the course where I was to make up for the time I'd lost, I was depleted physically and emotionally.

Was it the wall? It was hard to recognize. We hadn't seen each other in years.

Sometimes I think life is just making the same mistakes over again. For months I practiced positive self-talk and mental toughness in my workouts. And it worked. But when the chips were down in a race for which I'd so diligently prepared, I resorted to trash-talking myself and making excuses instead.

"But you finished," so many people will say, gently consoling me for what I describe as a poor performance.

I did finish; this is true. And at least I never walked.

Weather has been a factor in many of the most memorable Boston Marathons, from the searing heat of the 1976 "run for the hoses" to the Duel in the Sun standoff between Dick Beardsley and Alberto Salazar in 1982. Today's terrible conditions certainly contributed to unlikely outcomes.

Sarah Sellers, a nurse from Arizona who paid her own entry fee, came in behind winner Des Linden, shocked to take second place ahead of dozens of professionals who started the race in front of her. Likewise, Yuki Kawauchi, an unsponsored journeyman marathoner beloved in his native Japan, became the men's champion, despite lining up against men with personal records light-years ahead of his. Meanwhile, two-thirds of the elite field dropped out.

Unpredictable and sub-optimal weather isn't just a possibility at the Boston Marathon—it is among the race's defining characteristics. More than 4,000 registered runners elected not even to start in the weather today, which race organizers are now saying is the worst cold weather the Boston Marathon has seen in thirty years. Simply by enduring it, I earned my stripes, those three parallel lines on Boylston Street.

The race packets for the 2014 Boston Marathon contained bracelets made from banners that lined the course in 2013. The banners were cut up to make the bracelets, so no two are exactly alike. Each banner features a previous Boston Marathon champion or other notable race participants. Before that race, I wondered who was on the banner that became my bracelet. Today, four years later, I know it doesn't matter. It never did.

For years I behaved as if qualifying for and running the Boston Marathon would make me legitimate. I looked at the race from the outside, never realizing I was always already in it.

MARATHONS TO DATE

2004 Portland Marathon	4:23:23
2005 Seafair Marathon	4:13:07
2006 Vancouver Marathon	4:17:02
2006 Seattle Marathon	4:19:49
2007 Portland Marathon	3:59:06
2008 Eugene Marathon	3:57:00
2008 Portland Marathon	3:55:27
2009 Rock 'n' Roll Arizona Marathon	3:54:40
2009 Victoria Marathon	3:51:54
2010 Eugene Marathon	3:44:19
2010 Portland Marathon	4:19:09
2011 Boston Marathon	4:03:07
2012 Eugene Marathon	3:40:40
2013 Boston Marathon	3:41:27
2014 Boston Marathon	3:46:30
2016 New York Marathon	3:52:21
2017 Light at the End of the Tunnel Marathon	3:37:25
2018 Boston Marathon	4:13:22

Personal Best Times

Marathon	3:37:25 (2017)
Half Marathon	1:43:01 (2013)
5K	22:22 (2014)

ACKNOWLEDGMENTS

Writing a book is a lot like running a marathon, and Ronnie Alvarado and the team at Skyhorse Publishing are the best coaches this first-timer could've hoped for. I thank them for seeing the potential in my book proposal and helping me achieve it.

I'm grateful, too, for those who were with me at the start line; my earliest model of endurance, Olga Walker; Rosette Royale, who saw a story in my injury and suggested I begin writing it; and Jose Bautista, who encouraged me to keep putting one word in front of the other.

Enid Moore's passion for the Boston Marathon is contagious, and without her enthusiasm, I likely wouldn't be the runner—or writer—I am today.

Lily Unk and Melissa Frank-Huff showed me that grueling and exhilarating are two sides of the same workout. I thank them for inspiring me to take bigger strides—at the track, and on the page.

Whether it's a memoir or a marathon, getting to the finish line takes resilience, a trait epitomized by Bert Chavez and Glen Moore. For their example, and their friendship, I feel so fortunate.

Finally, I'm grateful to my family, for their love and support, especially my husband, Daniel Liberator, who has been my tailwind every step of the way.